MEDICAL
INTELLIGENCE
UNIT

HEART AND LUNG
TRANSPLANTATION 2000

Michael P. Kaye, M. D.

Minneapolis, Minnesota

John B. O'Connell, M. D.

University of Mississippi
Jackson, Mississippi

R.G. LANDES COMPANY
AUSTIN

MEDICAL INTELLIGENCE UNIT

HEART AND LUNG TRANSPLANTATION 2000

R.G. LANDES COMPANY
Austin / Georgetown

CRC Press is the exclusive worldwide distributor of publications of the Medical Intelligence Unit. CRC Press, 2000 Corporate Blvd., NW, Boca Raton, FL 33431. Phone: 407/994-0555.

Production Manager: Judith Kemper
Copy Editor: Constance Kerkaporta

Please address all inquiries to the Publisher:
R.G. Landes Company
909 South Pine Street
Georgetown, TX 78626
or
P.O. Box 4858
Austin, TX 78765
Phone: 512/ 863 7762
FAX: 512/ 863 0081

ISBN 1-879702-33-9
CATALOG # LN0233

INTRODUCTION

Over the past 25 years, heart transplantation and lung transplantation have evolved from the realm of science fiction, spearheaded by pioneering surgeons, to a widely applied modality for the treatment of end-stage heart disease. During this time, new immunosuppressive agents, endomyocardial biopsy and improved techniques of organ preservation have developed. However, impediments to continued growth and wider applicability have emerged because estimates of need far exceed the supply of donor organs as described in the opening chapter of this monograph by Dr. Roger Evans. Unfortunately, chronic rejection manifested as obliterative bronchiolitis in the lung and allograft vasculopathy in the heart has become the major limiting factor for long term survival as discussed by Tolman et al, Stuart and Baumgartner and Zerbe. Consequently, the need for retransplantation has increased.

In this text, Dr. David Cooper discusses the adverse neurohormonal cardiovascular effects of brain death and focuses on organ preservation. Dr. Thomas Egan summarizes lung donor selection and management and predicts various strategies to improve availability of lung donors. Dr. Sharon Hunt discusses areas that have frequently been overlooked, quality of life and functional rehabilitation after heart transplantation, and emphasizes the necessity of well designed quality of life trials. Dr. Maria-Teresa Olivari discusses an area that has been very frustrating, the accurate noninvasive diagnosis of cardiac allograft rejection. Similarly, Scott and Wallwork discuss noninvasive detection of pulmonary allograft rejection focusing on immune activation markers. Until immunosuppression becomes allograft-specific, infectious complications will remain a problem. Dr. Stephen Dummer provides insight into new technology and new approaches to the treatment and prevention of these serious infections. Dr. Jeffrey Hosenpud specifically addresses the problem of viral infections and provides a detailed discussion of new technologies and future approaches. Renlund et al discuss several new immunosuppressive agents and focus on their potential benefits. Dr. Daniel Salomon discusses novel approaches to target immune interaction with the allograft.

The indications for heart transplantation have changed dramatically in the last 25 years and one of the major advances has included the ability to perform cardiac transplantation on neonates. Chiavarelli and Bailey summarize the results and difficulties with neonatal transplantation.

As we enter the third millennium, alternatives to heart and lung replacement must be sought as discussed by McGary et al, Reichenspurner and Reichart. Novick et al review the serious problem of pulmonary preservation and predict directions for the future.

The purpose of this monograph is to update the reader on the current state of the art and speculate regarding the scientific accomplishments that will improve the effectiveness of thoracic organ replacement.

The authors would like to thank each of the contributors for their scholarly efforts and the outstanding secretarial support required to complete this text.

Michael P. Kaye, M.D.

John B. O'Connell, M.D.

CONTRIBUTORS

Leonard L. Bailey, M.D.
Loma Linda University Medical Center
Loma Linda, California

William A. Baumgartner, M.D.
Johns Hopkins Hospital
Baltimore, Maryland

Michael R. Bristow M.D., Ph. D.
University of Colorado
Health Sciences Center
Denver, Colorado

Mario Chiavarelli, M.D.
Loma Linda University Medical Center
Loma Linda, California

D.K.C. Cooper M.A., M.D., Ph.D., F.R.C.S.
Oklahoma Transplantation Institute
Baptist Medical Center
Oklahoma City, Oklahoma

Stephen Dummer, M.D.
Department of Medicine, Surgery and
Transplant Center
Vanderbilt University School of Medicine
Nashville, Tennessee

Thomas M. Egan, M.D., M.Sc.
Division of Cardiothoracic Surgery
University of North Carolina at Chapel Hill
Chapel Hill, North Carolina

R. Douglas Ensley, M.D.
Division of Cardiology
University of Utah Medical Center
Salt Lake City, Utah

Roger W. Evans, Ph.D.
Department of Health Sciences Research
Rochester, Minnesota

Michael L. Hess, M.D.
Medical College of Virginia
Virginia Commonwealth University
Richmond, Virginia

Jeffrey D. Hosenpud, M.D.
Oregon Cardiac Transplant Program
Portland, Oregon

Sharon A. Hunt, M.D.
Cardiac Transplant Program
Stanford University
Stanford, California

Suzan A. McGary, M.D.
Department of Surgery
Pennsylvania State University
Milton S. Hershey Medical Center
Hershey, Pennsylvania

F. Neil McKenzie, M.B., Ch.B., M.D.,
F.R.C.S.(E), F.R.C.S.(C)
Division of Cardiovascular-Thoracic Surgery
University Hospital
London, Ontario, Canada

Alan H. Menkis, M.D., F.R.C.S.(C)
Division of Cardiovascular-Thoracic Surgery
University Hospital
London, Ontario, Canada

P.K. Mohanty, M.D.
Department of Medicine
Medical College of Virginia
Virginia Commonwealth University
Richmond, Virginia

Richard J. Novick, M.D., M.Sc., F.R.C.S.(C),
F.A.C.S.
Division of Cardiovascular-Thoracic Surgery
University Hospital
London, Ontario, Canada

Maria-Teresa Olivari, M.D.
Division of Cardiology
Cardiac Transplant Program
The University of Texas Southwestern
Medical Center at Dallas
Dallas, Texas

Stephanie L. Olsen, M.D.
Division of Cardiology
University of Utah Medical Center
Salt Lake City, Utah

William S. Pierce, M.D.
Department of Surgery
Milton S. Hershey Medical Center
Pennsylvania State University
Hershey, Pennsylvania

Reed D. Quinn, M.D.
Department of Surgery
Pennsylvania State University
Milton S. Hershey Medical Center
Hershey, Pennsylvania

Bruno Reichart, M.D.
Department of Cardiac Surgery
Klinikum Grosshadern
University of Munich
Munich, Germany

Hermann Reichenspurner, M.D.
Department of Cardiac Surgery
Klinikum Grosshadern
University of Munich
Munich, Germany

Dale G. Renlund, M.D.
Division of Cardiology
University of Utah Medical Center
Salt Lake City, Utah

Daniel R. Salomon, M.D.
National Institutes of Health
Bethesda, Maryland

John P. Scott, M.D.
Papworth Hospital
Heart-Lung Transplant Unit
Cambridge, England

R. Scott Stuart, M.D.
Johns Hopkins Hospital
Baltimore, Maryland

Peter D. Taylor, M.D.
Department of Medicine
Medical College of Virginia
Virginia Commonwealth University
Richmond, Virginia

David E. Tolman, M.D.
Medical College of Virginia
Virginia Commonwealth University
Richmond, Virginia

John Wallwork, M.B., Ch.B., M.A., F.R.C.S.
Papworth Hospital
Cambridge, Enland

Tony R. Zerbe, M.D.
Presbyterian-University Hospital
of Pittsburgh
Pittsburgh, Pennsylvania

CONTENTS

CHAPTER 1

SOCIAL, ECONOMIC AND INSURANCE ISSUES IN HEART TRANSPLANTATION

Roger W. Evans

INTRODUCTION

Heart transplantation remains one of the most remarkable achievements in modern medicine. Initially considered a bold experiment, heart transplantation is now established therapy for a variety of end-stage cardiac diseases.[1-5] Foremost among these have been idiopathic cardiomyopathy and ischemic heart disease.[6] However, the procedure is not exclusively applied to adults, as children with congenital heart defects, particularly hypoplastic left heart syndrome, have benefitted from transplantation.[7-9]

Figure 1 shows the remarkable growth over the past decade in the number of heart transplants performed annually in the United States.[10] Coinciding with this substantial activity has been an unusually rapid increase in the number of transplant programs nationwide.[10] (Fig.2) This, in turn, has constrained, to some extent, the level of activity of all transplant centers, as shown in Figure 3.[10]

Despite its success, there has been much criticism of heart transplantation.[11-14] Critics contend that the procedure is excessively expensive, given other health care needs, and, in doing so, point to the size of the uninsured population in the United States, currently estimated at between 35 and 40 million people.[15,16] While such criticism has some validity, it is apparent that, on the basis of cost-per-year-of-life-gained, heart transplantation is no more expensive than a variety of currently accepted health care technologies and approaches to the treatment of catastrophic disease, including cancer.[17-21] Nonetheless, it is important to grasp the larger picture, and to consider the implications of heart transplantation in an era when health care technology is more likely to be criticized than admired. Just how heart transplantation will be regarded in this decade is clearly a matter of speculation. What is clear, however, is that the medical community will not stand alone when it comes to deciding how this technology will be used. The loudest voices are likely to be those of bureaucrats, health care policy makers, medical ethicists, lawyers, insurers, and patients themselves.

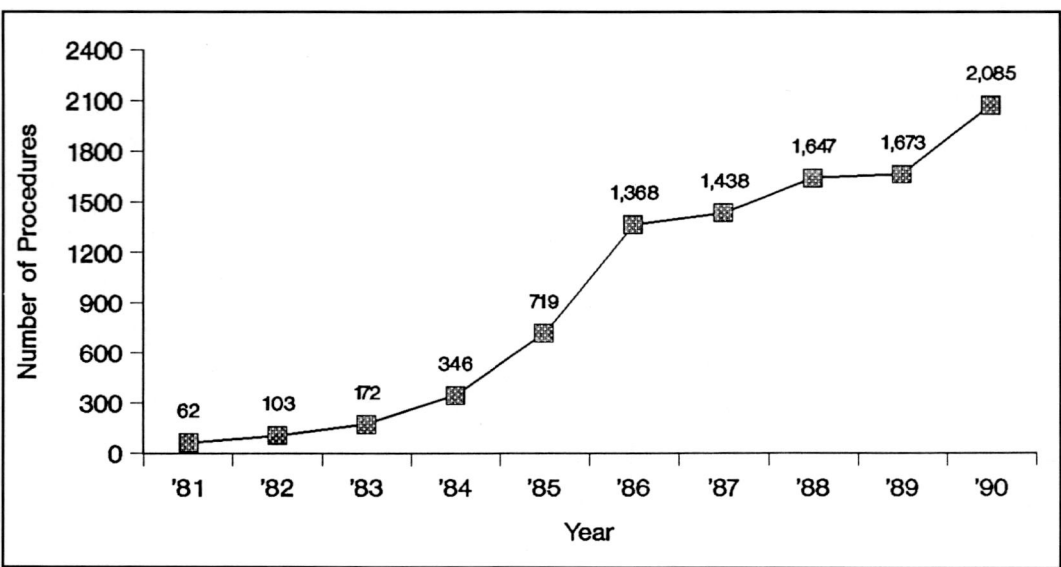

Fig. 1. Total number of heart transplants by year: 1981-1990.

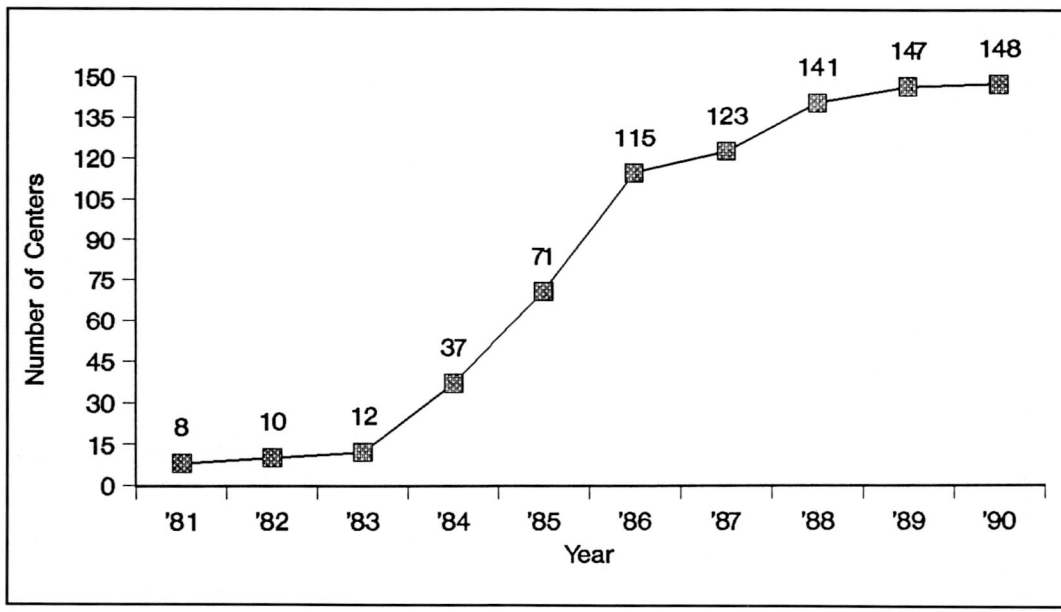

Fig. 2. Number of heart transplant programs in the U.S.: 1981-1990.

Differences of opinion may well serve to shape a controversial era in cardiology and cardiac surgery.

THE NEED AND DEMAND FOR HEART TRANSPLANTATION

The need for heart transplantation is considerable.[22] As patient selection criteria have become more liberal, need estimates, as de-picted in Figure 4, have increased substantially.[23-28] Based upon the most recently available mortality data, and an age criterion of 65 years, over 40,000 people die annually of conditions for which heart transplantation is indicated. However, as shown in Figure 5, age- and population-adjusted estimates indicate that, for persons between the ages of less than one-year through 65 years, and ages less

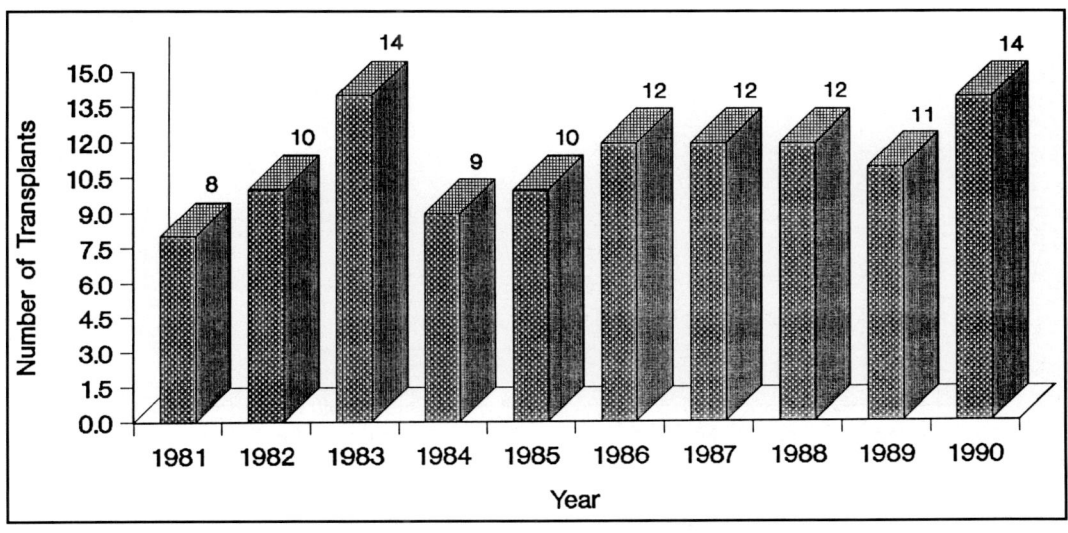

Fig. 3. Average number of heart transplants per center: 1981-1990.

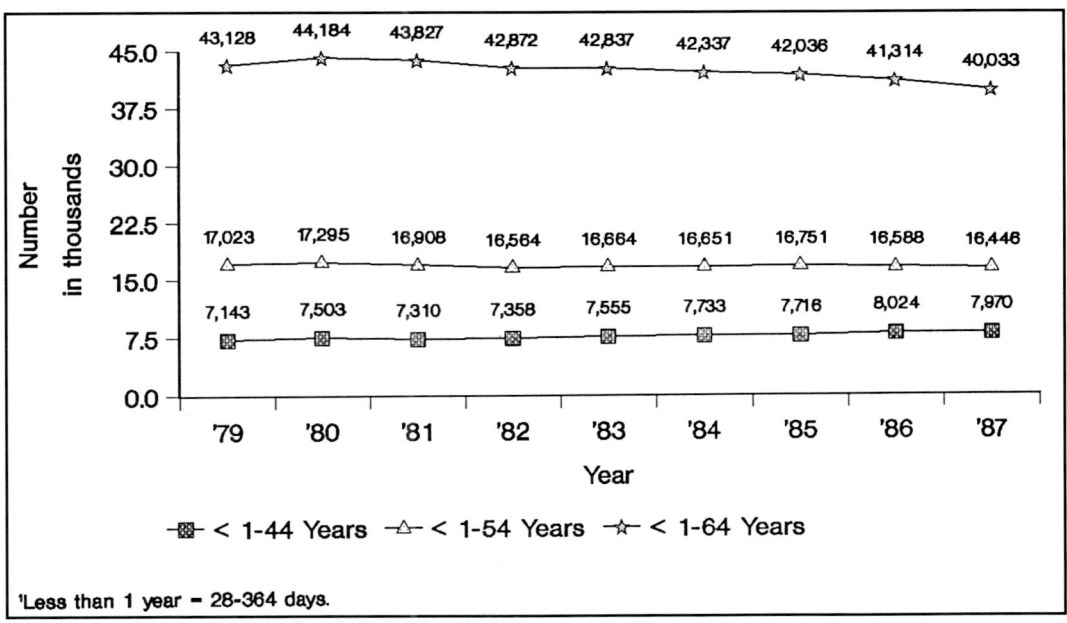

Fig. 4. Need for heart transplantation, 1979-87. (Number of persons)

than one-year through 55 years, there has actually been a decrease in deaths for which heart transplantation may be indicated. For persons between the ages of less than one-year through 45 years, there has been little change in mortality.

The demand for heart transplantation is an entirely different matter.[29] As shown in Figure 6, since December 1987 through June 1991, there has been a 2,296% increase in the number of persons awaiting heart transplantation. As these data suggest, an upward trend can be expected to continue as more people who could benefit from heart transplantation are referred to cardiologists for consideration. This pattern is likely to continue and to stimulate interest in transplantation, perhaps encouraging additional hospitals to initiate new

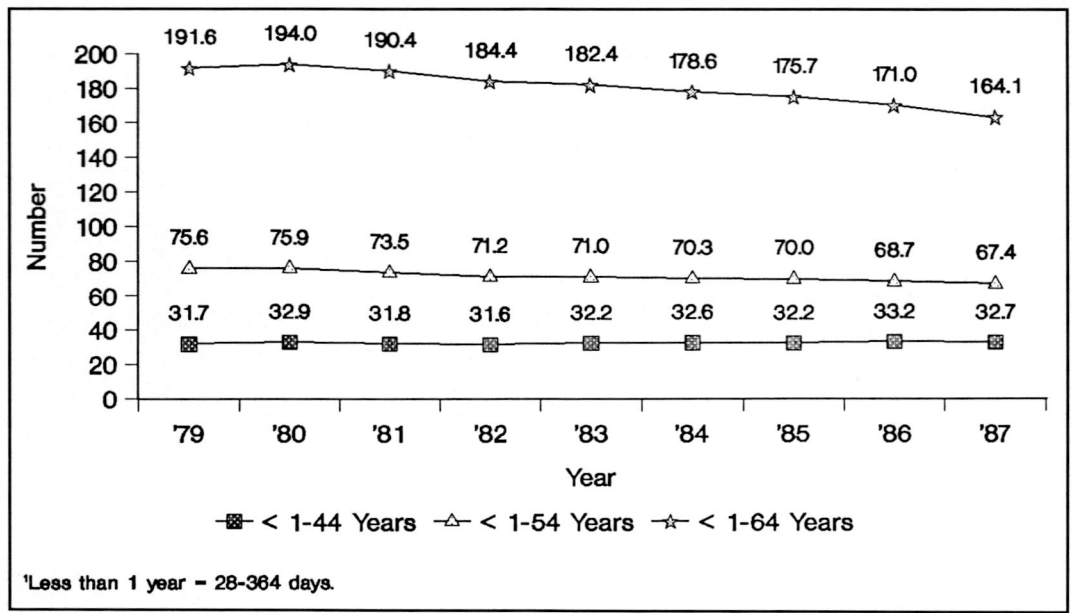

Fig. 5. Need for heart transplantation, 1979-87. (per million population)

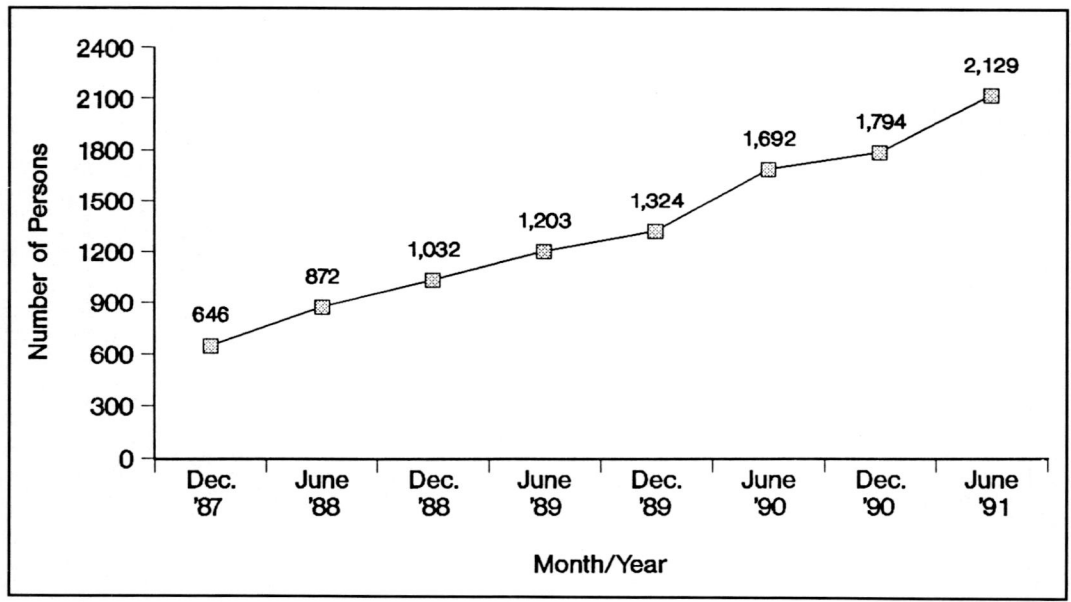

Fig. 6. UNOS heart transplant waiting list: December, 1987—June, 1991.

programs.[30-35] Due to a limited supply of donor hearts, this may be an unwise administrative decision, particularly in geographic areas currently served by one or more heart transplant programs.[36-42]

ORGAN DONOR SUPPLY

The primary constraint on all transplant activity has been an inadequate supply of donor organs. Figure 7 provides a summary of the number of organ donors in the United

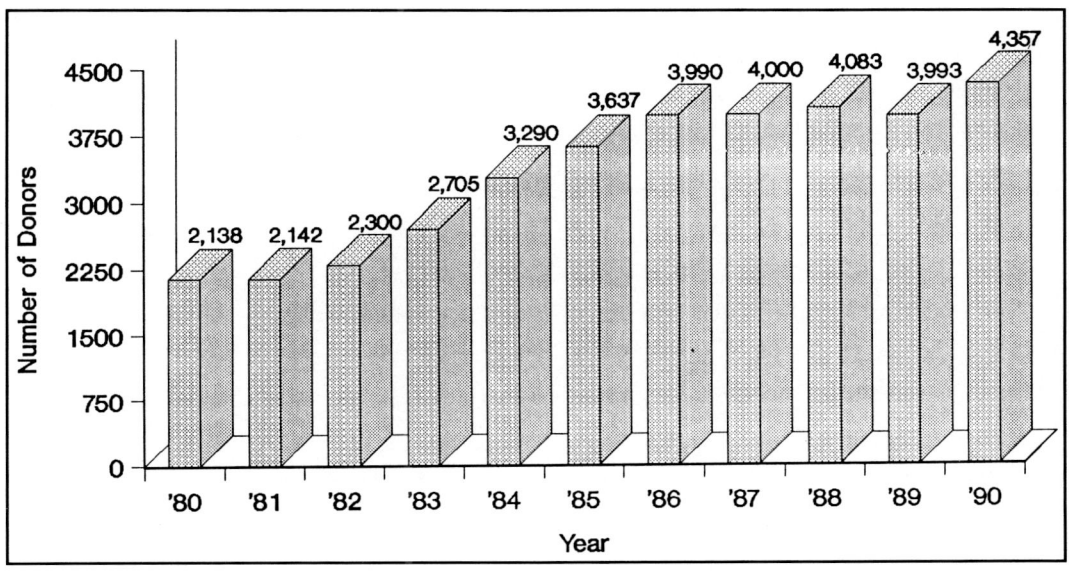

Fig. 7. Estimated number of organ donors by year: 1980-1990.

States for the period 1980-1990.[36,37] As shown, between 1986 and 1989 there were approximately 4,000 donors annually. While there was a slight increase in 1990, this may simply reflect the tendency to use more liberal criteria for donor selection.[43,44] In other words, if donor criteria were held constant over time, it is unlikely that the supply of donors has changed. If anything, the number of criteria-adjusted donors may actually have decreased.

Of course, not every organ donor is the source of a suitable heart. Heart donor criteria remain among the more stringent in use today.[5] Based upon actual transplant activity, in 1990, about 47.9% of all donors were the source of an acceptable heart.

Over the years there has been much speculation as to the size of the potential donor pool.[36,37,42] Numerous estimates are summarized in Table 1. As shown, the majority of recent studies suggest that approximately 10,000 donors may be available annually. A point estimate of 7,300 donors is perhaps most realistic, based upon recently completed research.[37] Clearly, the data summarized here suggest that the supply of donor hearts is unlikely to be satisfactory to meet demand, given the actual need for heart transplantation.

THE BENEFITS OF HEART TRANSPLANTATION

Although the social and political challenges faced by transplantation specialists are considerable, the benefits that patients derive are noteworthy.[45,46] Figure 8 summarizes survival data from the Registry of the International Society for Heart and Lung Transplantation for both heterotopic and orthotopic transplantation.[47] The results of orthotopic transplantation exceed those of heterotopic transplantation, but the latter procedure is rarely performed.

Achievements related to patient survival are even more remarkable, considering the data from Stanford University Medical Center summarized in Table 2.[48] As shown, one-year patient survival improved from 22% in 1968 to 83% in 1983.

Patient quality of life has also improved over the past two decades.[45] It is currently estimated that between 32 and 50% of heart transplant recipients actually return to work, although nearly 60% report that they are able to do so. Both patient preference and employer discrimination play a significant role in the return to work decision of many patients. Patients who have been spared from death do not always consider return to work

Table 1. Estimates of Potential Donor Supply

Area Studied	Year	Donors[1] P.M.P.	National[2] Estimate of Donors
Georgia	1975 1976-79	43.0 - 55.0	10,700 - 14,000
Georgia, Kansas, Missouri	1975	55.0 - 116.0	14,000 - 29,000
Varies by Study	1986	68.0 - 104.0	17,000 - 26,000
Pennsylvania	1987	38.3 - 55.2	10,000 - 14,000
Kentucky	1989	48.0	12,000
Rhode Island, Vermont (2 States)	1990	20.0 - 40.0	5,000 - 10,000
United States	1991	28.5 - 43.7	6,900 - 10,700

[1]PMP = per million population.
[2]Based upon 249.6 million official United States' population in 1990.
*Personal communication with Carl Haisch, M.D., University of Vermont, Burlington, Vermont.[36-37]

Table 2. Percentage of Patients Surviving One-Year Following Cardiac Transplantation at Stanford University Medical Center

Year of Transplantation	One-Year Survival
1968	22%
1972	54%
1977	58%
1983	83%

SOURCE: Reference 7, page 398.

as a foremost objective in their lives. For many patients, "living one day at a time" is hardly conducive to career planning.

Most heart transplant recipients—between 80 and 85%—are reported to be physically active and "fully rehabilitated."[45] In this context, rehabilitation refers to all aspects of major life activities, not just employment.

There are also critical subjective aspects which must be considered in any attempt to evaluate the quality of life of transplant recipients.[45,46] Among the more critical indicators are well-being, life satisfaction, and psychological effect. Figures 9, 10, and 11 provide a comparative assessment of the subjective quality of life of a variety of different types of transplant recipients. As shown, on most indicators, there is relatively little difference between the recipients of various transplants and the general population of the United States (denoted as GPOP).

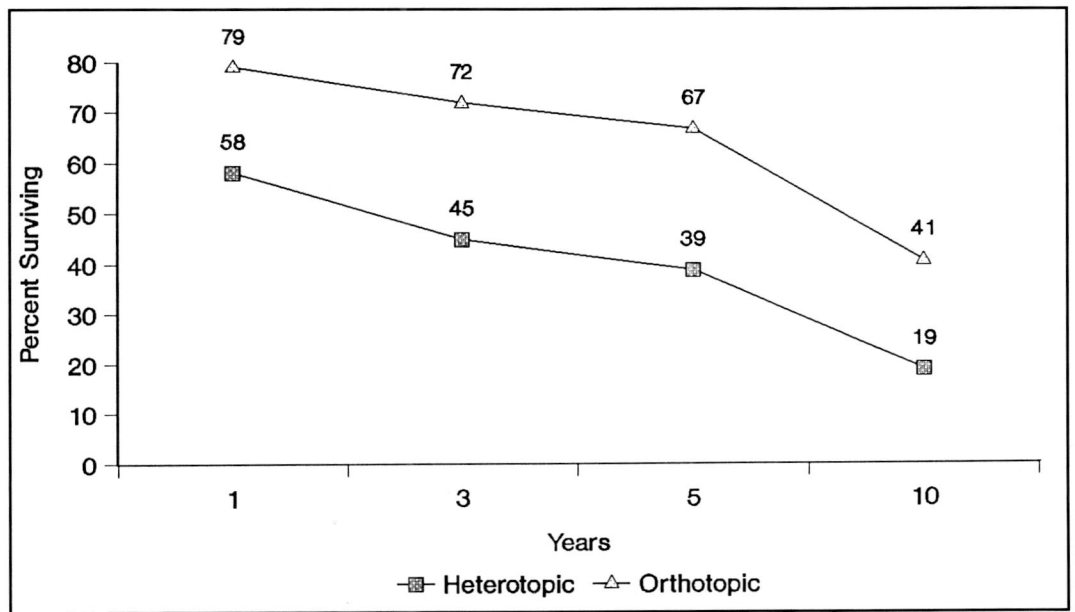

Fig. 8. Heart transplant patient survival rates.

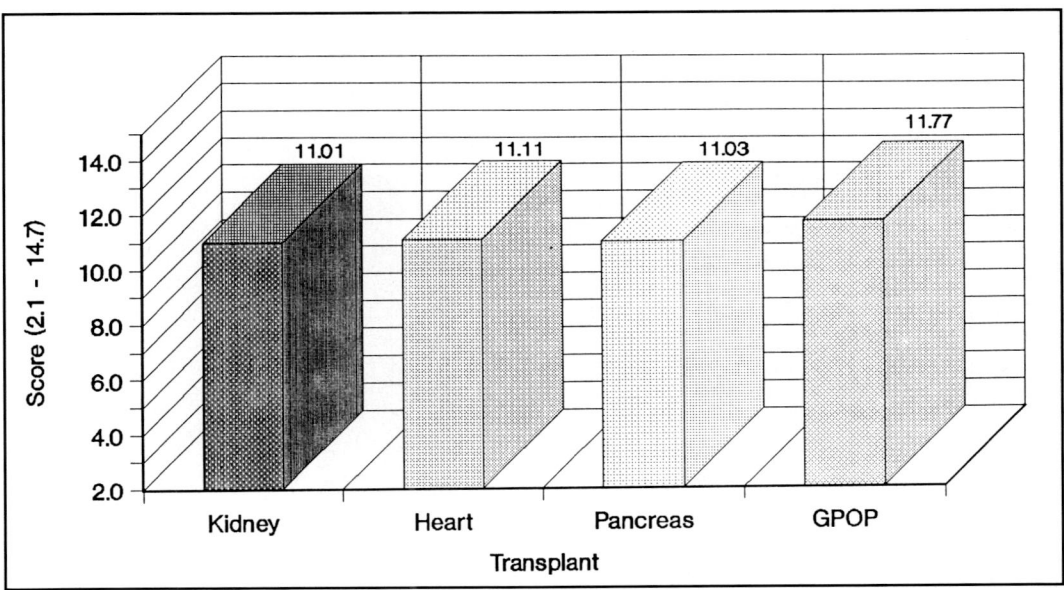

Fig. 9. Well-being by transplant procedure.

Despite the quality of their lives, many heart transplant recipients experience difficulties reintegrating themselves into the society of which they are a part. Often psychological and psychiatric disturbances are manifested and, as a result, the support of appropriate mental health professionals must be sought. Not all patients are equally adept at meeting the rigors of the therapeutic regimen associated with transplantation therapy. Because of these problems, and what some critics regard as a compromised quality of life, the cost of heart transplantation has become the subject of an ever-increasingly emotional debate.

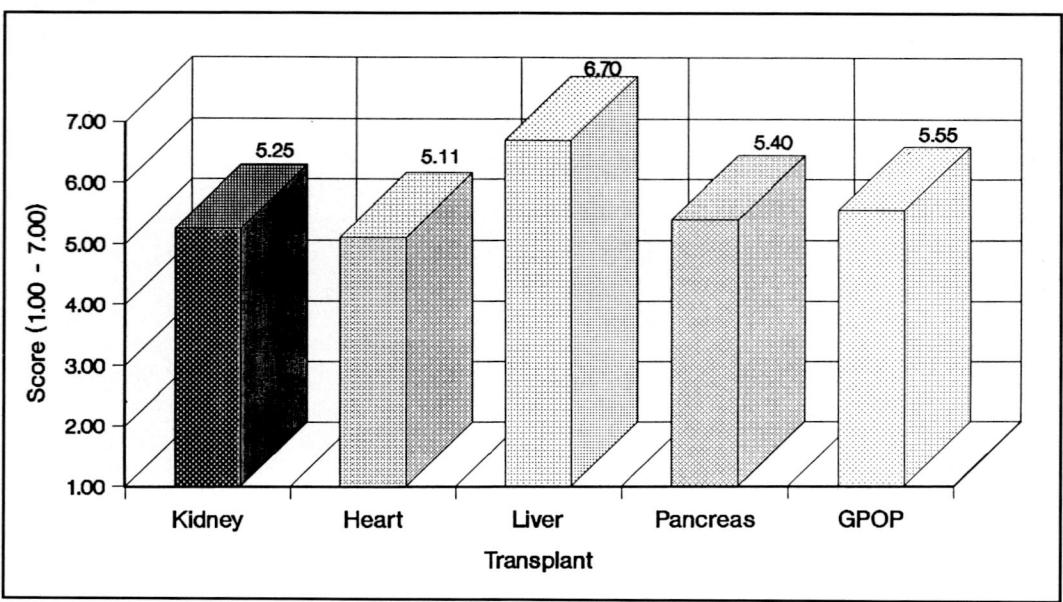

Fig. 10. Life satisfaction by transplant procedure.

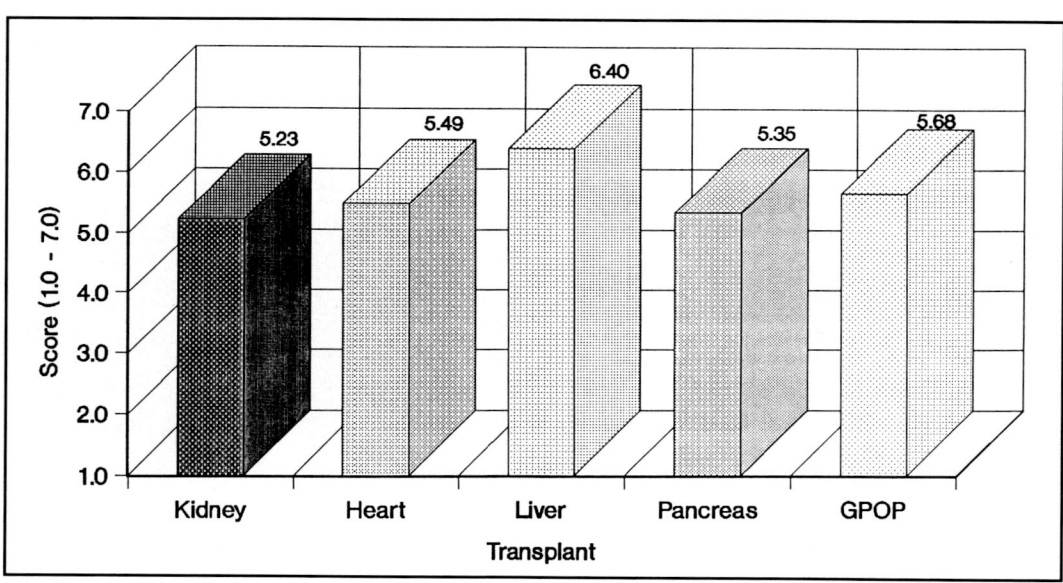

Fig. 11. Psychological effect of transplant procedure.

THE COST OF HEART TRANSPLANTATION

The cost of heart transplantation has recently been examined in detail in the National Cooperative Transplantation Study (NCTS).[5,14,49] Procedure charges were carefully assessed for kidney, heart, liver, heart-lung, and pancreas transplantation.[5,49] The overall results are presented in Figure 12, which shows total charges incurred from date of transplant until initial hospital discharge. The estimated ranges of procedure-specific charges are summarized in Table 3. Finally, a breakdown of each heart transplant element of charge, including hospital

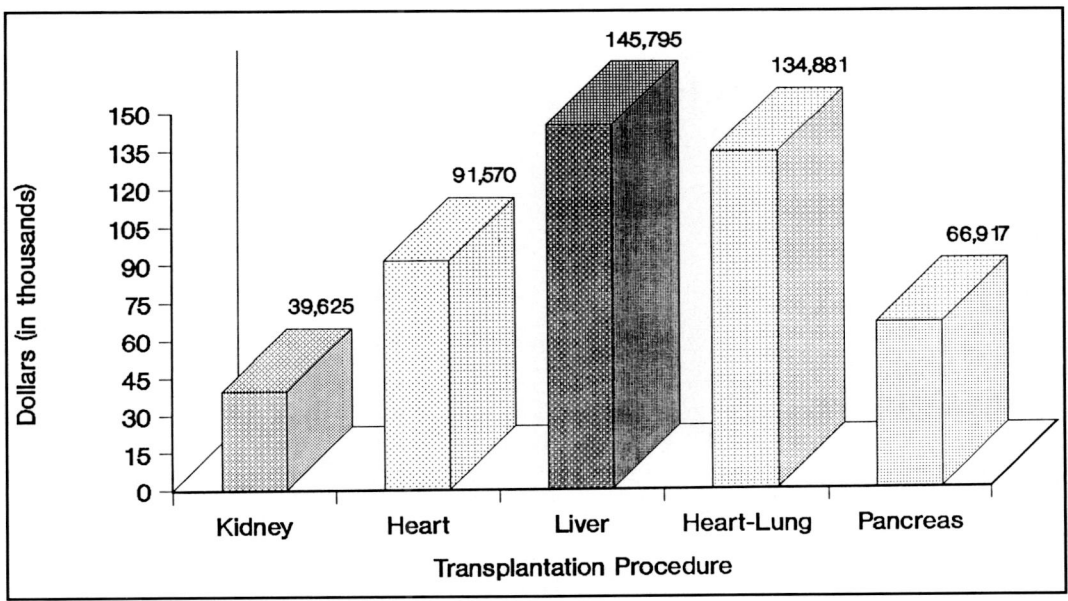

Fig. 12. Median transplantation procedure charges, 1988.

Table 3. Range of Transplantation Procedure Charges, 1988

	Range		
Transplant	Low	High	Median
Kidney	$ 7,573	$ 622,903	$ 39,625
Heart	10,725	1,465,640	91,570
Liver	32,028	1,622,544	145,776
Heart-Lung	56,105	461,862	134,881
Pancreas	15,818	573,605	66,917

SOURCE: Reference 5.

charges, surgeons' fees, other professional fees, and donor organ acquisition charges, is provided in Figure 13.[14] As shown, on average, a heart transplant procedure costs $91,570 with an average length of hospital stay of 23 days. However, as depicted in Table 3, above, there is considerable variation in the charges associated with all transplant procedures.[5,49]

It is of interest to note that, adjusted for inflation, the average cost of a heart transplant has decreased. Table 4 presents inflation-adjusted heart transplantation charge data based upon the National Heart Transplantation Study (NHTS), completed in 1984.[1,21] Comparing the NCTS data with those of the NHTS, adjusting for inflation, shows a net decrease of $13,739 in heart transplant procedure charges. This, perhaps, is in large part due to a reduction in the average length of hospital stay, from 61 to 23 days.

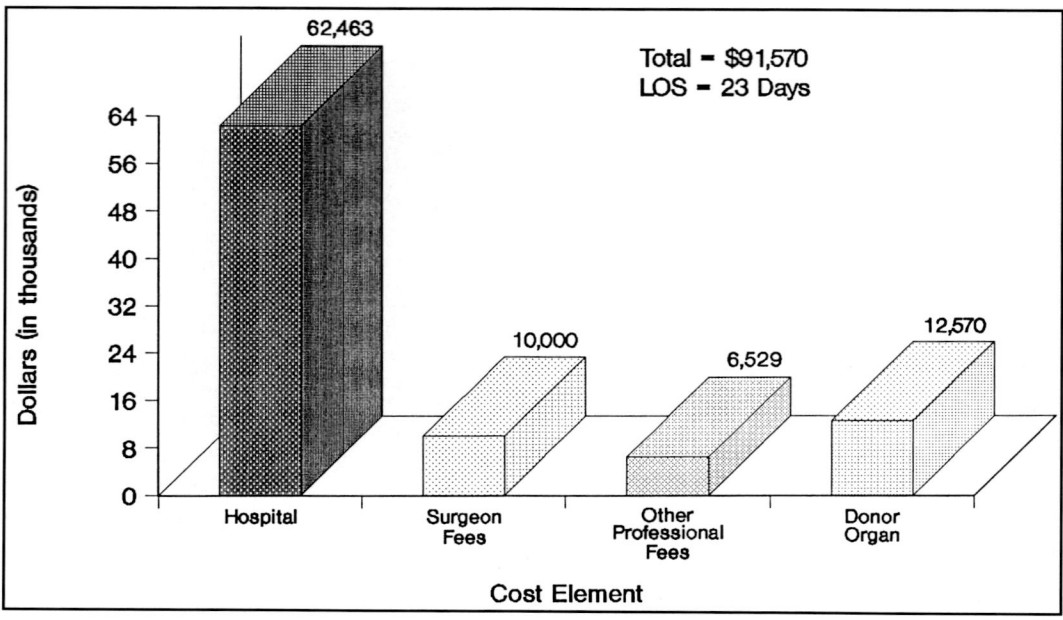

Fig. 13. Median heart transplantation procedure charges, 1988.

INSURANCE COVERAGE AND REIMBURSEMENT

Although insurance coverage for organ transplantation has improved steadily over the years, some significant problems still persist.[2-4,14,16,49] First, coverage per se does not guarantee an adequate level of reimbursement. In other words, while an insurer may pay for heart transplants, the amount they reimburse may be substantially below actual billed hospital charges. For example, although Medicare covers heart transplants for eligible beneficiaries, the amount paid is about 60% of billed charges. During the period 1985-90, average billed charges for a Medicare-covered heart transplant were $100,690, with an average reimbursement equal to $59,292.[14]

Medicare remains fairly restrictive in its coverage of heart transplants. It carefully defines eligible beneficiaries and restricts payment to "qualified" or approved providers. Currently, of the 148 heart transplant programs in the United States, only 47 are Medicare-approved.

Medicaid benefits are provided by individual states and involve Federal matching funds.[14,16] In other words, the Federal government, through the Health Care Financing Administration, partially subsidizes the Medicaid programs of all states at a level between 50 and 78%. Heart transplantation, however, is not a federally mandated benefit, but coverage has improved. In 1985, 49% of states (including the District of Columbia) offered coverage. This increased to 65% in 1986, 69% in 1988, and 78% in 1990.[14]

Private insurer coverage of organ transplants is difficult to track. Currently the best available

Table 4. Inflation-Adjusted Heart Transplantation Charges Based Upon the National Heart Transplantation Study

Year	Inflation Multiplier	Average Charge
1983	—	$ 76,435
1984	1.062	81,174
1985	1.063	86,288
1986	1.075	92,760
1987	1.066	98,882
1988	1.065	105,309

data are compiled by the Health Insurance Association of American (HIAA), the industry representative for commercial insurers.[3,4,14] Blue Cross and Blue Shield plans are independent organizations and are not members of the HIAA. In 1985, 55% of the major insurance companies represented by HIAA offered heart transplant coverage. In 1988, this percentage increased to 84%. More recent data are not yet available.

In assessing private insurer coverage of transplantation, it is important to keep in mind that, while an insurer may offer coverage for transplantation, employers who extend benefits to their employees may exclude certain transplantations as part of their standard benefit packages.[16] Therefore, the only way to truly know what fraction of people in the United States has coverage for heart transplantation would be to evaluate benefit packages at the level of the employer for each worker in the country. This would clearly be a difficult task to accomplish.

Of the heart transplants performed in 1988, 7% were paid for by Medicare, 6% by Medicaid, and the remainder, 87%, by other, predominantly private, insurers or sources.[50]

As noted above, an underrecovery of charges can be a problem for some transplantation centers. Based upon the National Cooperative Transplantation Study, in 11% of the cases examined, reimbursement of hospital charges was between 0 and 20%, 10% between 21 and 60%, and 7% between 61 and 80%.[50] In 72% of all cases, reimbursement equalled more than 80% of hospital charges.

A final comment concerns ability-to-pay and access to transplantation as a general matter.[15,50] Several studies have suggested that minorities do not have equal access to transplantation.[51-53] While this may be the case, it is unclear as to whether this is a race or an economic effect. It is clear, however, that the reimbursement of hospital charges is more favorable for privately insured as opposed to publicly insured patients. For example, in the case of heart transplantation, 80% or more of hospital charges were paid for 82% of privately insured patients, compared with 43% of patients without private insurance.[50] Since minorities are more likely to be publicly-insured, thus representing, to some extent, an economic liability to transplant centers, they may have a more difficult time meeting the economic and insurance requirements maintained by transplant programs which are anxious about cost recovery.

INSURER DESIGNATION OF TRANSPLANT CENTERS

In an effort to assure patients of the best possible outcome at an acceptable cost, many major health insurers have begun to designate transplant centers, restricting reimbursement to those programs that offer the highest quality of care.[54-58] The designation of centers is usually based upon criteria that emphasize experience, qualifications, and outcomes, of which in the latter instance, survival has been primary.[54] In return for volume referrals, insurers expect transplantation hospitals to negotiate favorable reimbursement rates. Some insurers claim to have received per procedure discounts of between 25 and 30%. Patients are encouraged by insurers to use designated providers on grounds that their transplantation is more likely to be successful when performed at a "center of excellence." As further inducement, some insurers offer a variety of incentives if a patient goes to a designated transplantation program, including coverage of travel costs for the patient as well as a family member, and increasing surgical benefits from 70 or 80% to 90 or 100%.

The designation of centers is typically based upon a triangular hypothesis linking volume with both costs and outcome.[54] In short, insurers have assumed that high volume manifests itself in better outcomes and lower costs. In addition, better outcomes are expected to be less costly than poor outcomes. Data from the National Cooperative Transplantation Study, presented in Tables 5 and 6, allow for a reasonable test of these hypotheses.[5,59] As shown in Table 5, there is little relationship between total transplant procedure charges and program volume, although the length of hospital stay for patients at low volume centers is five days longer than that of

Table 5. Heart Transplant Procedure Charges, Length of Hospital Stay, and Patient Outcome Based on Program Volume

Transplant Program Volume[1]	Total Procedure Charges (Dollars)	Length of Hospital Stay (Days)	One-Year Patient Survival (Percent)
Less than 12 Transplants	$ 89,731	27	80.2%
12-50 Transplants	91,068	22	83.4
Over 50 Transplants	90,855	22	80.6
Overall	$ 91,570	23	82.4%

[1]1988 only.
SOURCE: References 14 and 59.

patients transplanted at more active centers.[14,59] Also, as is apparent from Table 5, one-year patient survival has only a modest relationship with program volume. Patients transplanted at centers performing between 12 and 50 procedures have a slightly better outcome than that of patients transplanted at low and high volume centers. Finally, as shown in Table 6, poor outcomes—both death within one-month or death within one-year—are associated with higher initial transplant procedure charges. Thus, of the three hypotheses which serve as the basis for insurer designation of transplant centers, only one is confirmed by

Table 6. Heart Transplant Procedure Charges Based Upon Patient Survival at One-Month and One-Year

Survival Period	Total Procedure Charges (Dollars)	Length of Hospital Stay (Days)
Patient Survival (One-Month)		
Yes	$ 89,962	23
No	97,696	11
Patient Survival (One-Year)		
Yes	88,508	22
No	103,192	22
Overall	$ 91,570	23

SOURCE: Reference 14.

empirical data. This does not mean, however, that a heart transplant center effect is nonexistent. The center effect in heart transplantation is, quite simply, due to factors other than total program volume, as demonstrated in the National Cooperative Transplantation Study.[59,60]

Despite these results, it is likely that insurers will continue to subscribe to the transplant program experience rationale and, most likely, will continue to designate centers on the basis of minimum program volume and threshold survival results.[54] Table 7 summarizes the volume-outcome criteria for heart transplantation centers being used by public and private insurers today. It should also be emphasized that, while United Network for Organ Sharing membership is a necessary condition for designation, it is by no means a sufficient condition.

Finally, there is concern within the transplant community that some insurers are being devious in their efforts to designate transplant centers.[54] Despite the stated intentions of insurers, some transplant professionals

believe the ultimate objective of insurers is to inhibit access to transplantation, thereby limiting the number of transplants for which they pay. Thus far there is little evidence that access is a major problem, and some insurers have actually begun to increase the number of transplant centers participating in their networks. Perhaps a greater concern should lie with the adequacy of reimbursement transplant centers receive in return for procedures performed.

DISCUSSION

The data presented here raise a variety of sensitive issues, most of which are more easily discussed than resolved. The reasons for this are quite clear. For example, while the need for heart transplantation has begun to level-off, the demand for the procedure will continue to increase. However, even with incremental annual increases in donor supply, it is unlikely that a sufficient number of donor hearts will be available to meet demand. Thus, difficult questions will continue to be raised as to which patients constitute the most acceptable transplant recipients. If cost-effectiveness is used as the primary allocation principle, it is clear that many patients who are given priority for transplant will no longer be accorded this status. Not only do the sickest patients have the poorest outcomes, they also have higher per procedure transplant procedure charges.

In the absence of an adequate supply of donor hearts, both xenotransplantation and mechanical circulatory support systems must be reconsidered.[61-70] However, public support for these approaches is questionable, with the artificial heart program of the National Institutes of Health always in a state of uncertainty.[62] Health care policymakers now appear to reject the very concept of viable long-term mechanical option to heart transplantation. Both cost and quality of life considerations have contributed to public apathy. Many policymakers contend that if heart transplantation represents a misuse of scarce public resources, the artificial heart is a public policy nightmare society is better off without. Xenotransplantation has its own problems in light of animal rights concerns and aggressive attempts to limit the use of ani-

Table 7. Minimum Heart Transplantation Program Volume and Outcome Standards Specified by Selected Public and Private Health Insurers

Criterion	Program Value
Annual Volume (#)	
Pediatric	6
Adult	12-15
Overall	25
One-Year Survival (%)	
Pediatric	75%
Adult	80%
Overall	80-85%

SOURCE: Reference 54.

Table 8. The Costs and Outcomes of Mechanical Circulatory Support and Retransplantation

		Total Procedure Charges (Dollars)	Length of Hospital Stay (Days)	One-Year Patient Survival (Percent)
Mechanical Circulatory Support				
	Yes	$ 227,653	46	63.9
	No	88,108	22	83.3
Retransplantation				
	Yes	112,450	26	60.9
	No	89,394	22	83.3

SOURCE: Reference 14.

mals in research and experimentation.[68] Thus, there is now evidence that life has a price that exceeds both the willingness and ability of the public to pay. Death may be perceived as the preferred alternative to cardiac replacement.

The benefits of transplantation, although substantial, may not be sufficient to justify further expenditures.[71] As described here, the cost of transplantation is great, but not necessarily excessive, given the costs associated with the care of other catastrophically ill patients. There are, nonetheless, excesses which require careful scrutiny. These include the use of mechanical devices as a bridge to transplant and retransplantation. Data summarized in Table 8 reveal the economic and survival consequences of these interventions. Clearly, costs can be great and outcomes poor, calling into question the cost-effectiveness of these treatment approaches.

Insurers have adapted remarkably well to the economic consequences of heart transplantation. The concept of designating transplant centers is heuristic although, in some instances, this may create personal hardships for some patients who must travel great distances to a designated provider.[54,58] Such travel is required at exactly that point in time when

patients are most vulnerable. Their survival hangs in the balance, their family may be at the point of despair, and then, making matters even more difficult, they come under the care of a transplant team with which they are unfamiliar. In some respects, the very survival of patients may be jeopardized in the referral process. While the goals of insurers are laudable, the needs of patients may be inadequately appreciated. All of this is to suggest that the designated-provider approach to the provision of transplantation services must, itself, be carefully monitored. While patient survival is the foremost concern, this could well be adversely affected through psychosocial vulnerability. Thus far, insurers have not developed research protocols to assess the consequences of designating providers.

Much uncertainty surrounds the future of heart transplantation. While there is now little disagreement as to the therapeutic advantages of heart transplantation over other treatment approaches, it is unclear exactly what level of benefit must be achieved to sustain enthusiasm for the procedure. As definitions of acceptability change in the face of economic constraint, the sociopolitical and socioeconomic challenges to heart transplantation could be grave. What is valued today could conceivably be discounted tomorrow. As a result, the objective will be to continue to both improve upon and demonstrate the clinical efficacy and economic acceptability of heart transplantation.

ACKNOWLEDGEMENT

This research was generously supported by the United Network for Organ Sharing and the Health Care Financing Administration. Word processing support was provided by Ms. June Hull and all graphic displays of data were prepared by Ms. Donna McLynne.

REFERENCES

1. Evans RW, Manninen DL, Overcast TD et al. The National Heart Transplantation Study: Final report. Seattle, WA Battelle Human Affairs Research Centers, 1984.
2. Evans RW. Coverage and reimbursement for heart transplantation. Int J of Technology Assessment in Health Care 1986; 2:425-449.
3. Evans RW. Third party payment and the cost of transplantation. J South Carolina Med Assoc 1991; 87:345-352.
4. Evans RW. Organ transplantation costs, insurance coverage and reimbursement. In: Terasaki PI, ed. Clinical Transplants, 1990. Los Angeles UCLA Tissue Typing Laboratory, 1990:343-355.
5. Evans RW, Manninen DL, Dong FB. The National Cooperative Transplantation Study: Final report. Seattle, WA Battelle-Seattle Research Center, June 1991.
6. Kriett JM, Kaye MP. The Registry of the International Society for Heart Transplantation: Seventh official report—1990. J. Heart Transplant 1990; 9:323-330.
7. Bailey LL, Wood M, Razzouk A, Van Arsdell G, Gundry S. Heart transplantation during the first 12 years of life. Arch Surg 1989; 124:1221-1226.
8. Starnes VA, Bernstein D, Oyer PE et al. Heart transplantation in children. J Heart Transplant 1989; 8:20-26.
9. Stuart AG, Wren C, Sharples PM, Hunter S, Hey EN. Hypoplastic left heart syndrome: More potential transplant recipients than suitable donors. Lancet 1991; 337:957-959.
10. Evans RW. Organ transplantation activity in the United States. In: Evans RW, Manninen DL, Dong FB., eds. The National Cooperative Transplantation Study: Final Report. Seattle Battelle-Seattle Research Center, 1991.
11. Baily MA. Economic issues in organ substitution policy. In: Mathieu D, ed. Organ Substitution Technology. Boulder: Westview Press, 1988:198-210.
12. Evans RW. The private sector vis-a-vis the government in future funding of organ transplantation. Transplant Proc 1990; 22:975-979.
13. Dean M. Is your treatment economic, effective, efficient? Lancet 1991; 337(8739):480-481.
14. Evans RW, Manninen DL, Dong FB. Costs, insurance coverage, and reimbursement for heart transplantation. In: Evans RW, Manninen DL, Dong FB, eds. The National Cooperative Transplantation Study: Final Report. Seattle: Battelle-Seattle Research Center, June 1991.
15. Evans RW. Money matters: Should ability to pay ever be a consideration in gaining access to transplantation? Transplant Proc 1989; 21:3419-3423.
16. Evans RW. Insurance coverage and reimbursement for transplantation. In: Evans RW, Manninen DL, Dong FB,eds. The National Cooperative Transplantation Study: Final Report. Seattle: Battelle-Seattle Research Center, 1991.
17. Evans RW. The socioeconomics of organ transplantation. Transplant Proc 1985; 17(6) Suppl 4:129-136.
18. Evans RW. The heart transplant dilemma. Issues in Science and Technology 1986; 2(3):91-101.
19. Evans RW. Cost effectiveness analysis of transplantation. Surg Clinics of North America. 1986; 66:603-616.
20. Evans RW. A catastrophic disease perspective on organ transplantation. In: Ginzberg E, ed. Medicine and Society: Clinical Decisions and Societal Values. Boulder: Westview Press, 1987:61-95.
21. Evans RW. The economics of heart transplantation. Circulation 1987; 75:63-76.
22. Evans RW, Orians CE. The need for transplantation in the United States. In: Evans RW, Manninen DL, Dong FB, eds. The National Cooperative Transplantation Study: Final report. Seattle: Battelle-Seattle Research Center, 1991.
23. Carrier M, Emery RW, Riley JE, Levinson MM, Copeland JG. Cardiac transplantation in patients over 50 years of age. J Am Coll Cardiol 1986; 8:285-288.
24. McAleer-Rhenman MJ, Rhenman B, Icenogle TB et al. Diabetes mellitus in heart transplantation. J Heart Transplant 1988; 7:64.
25. Miller LW, Vitale-Noedel N, Pennington G, McBride L, Kanter KR. Heart transplantation in patients over age fifty-five years. J Heart Transplant 1988; 7:254-257.
26. Olivari MT, Antolick A, Kaye MP, Jamieson SW, Ring WS. Heart transplantation in elderly patients. J Heart Transplant 1988; 7:258-264.
27. Armitage JM, Kormos RL, Griffith BP et al. Heart transplantation in patients with malignant disease. J Heart Transplant 1990; 9:627-630.
28. Ladowski JS, Kormos RL, Uretsky BP, Griffith BP, Armitage JM, Hardesty RL. Heart transplantation in diabetic recipients. Transplantation 1990; 49:303-305.
29. Evans RW. The demand for transplantation in the United States. In: Terasaki PI, ed. Clinical Trans-

plants, 1990. Los Angeles: UCLA Tissue Typing Laboratory, 1990:319-327.

30. Moore FD. How much cardiac transplantation—and where? Heart Transplantation 1982; 1:254-256.

31. English TAH. Presidential address. J Heart Transplant 1984; 4:12.

32. Copeland JG. Presidential address: Facts to be considered prior to undertaking a heart transplantation program. Heart Transplantation 1984; 3:275-277.

33. Losman JG. Too many and not enough. J Heart Transplant 1985; 4:282.

34. Russell PS. Centers for transplantation—how many should we have? Surgery 1986; 100(5):867-876.

35. Monaco AP. Problems in transplantation—ethics, education, expansion. Transplantation 1987; 43:1-4.

36. Evans RW. The actual and potential supply of organ donors in the United States. In: Terasaki PI, ed. Clinical Transplants, 1990. Los Angeles: UCLA Tissue Typing Laboratory, 1990:329-341.

37. Evans RW, Orians CE, Ascher NL. The potential supply of organ donors: An assessment of the efficiency of organ procurement efforts in the United States. JAMA 1992; 267:239-246.

38. Evans RW, Manninen DL, Garrison LP, Jr, Maier A. Donor availability as the primary determinant of the future of heart transplantation. JAMA 1986; 255:1892-1898.

39. Evans RW. Trauma registries and organ transplantation. JAMA 1990; 263:1913-1914.

40. Koop CE. Increasing the supply of solid organs for transplantation. Public Health Rep 1983; 98:566-572.

41. Gore SM, Taylor RMR, Wallwork J. Availability of transplantable organs from brain dead donors in intensive care units. Br Med J 1991; 302:149-153.

42. Nathan HM, Jarrell BE, Broznik B et al. Estimation and characterization of the potential renal organ donor pool in Pennsylvania: Report of the pennsylvania statewide donor study. Transplantation 1991; 51:142-149.

43. Alexander JW, Vaughn WK. The use of "marginal" donors for organ transplantation: The influence of age on outcome. Transplantation 1991; 51:135-141.

44. Alexander JW, Vaughn WK, Carery MA. The use of marginal donors for organ transplantation: The older and younger donors. Transplant Proc 1991; 23:905-909.

45. Evans RW. The benefits of transplantation. In: Evans RW, Manninen DL, Dong FB, eds. The National Cooperative Transplantation Study: Final report. Battelle-Seattle Research Center, June 1991.

46. Evans RW. Psychosocial aspects of heart transplantation: A comparative analysis. In: Evans RW, Manninen DL, Dong FB, eds. The National Cooperative Transplantation Study: Final report. Seattle: Battelle-Seattle Research Center, June 1991.

47. Kriett JM, Kaye MP. The registry of the international society for heart transplantation: Eighth official report—1991. J Heart Lung Transplant 1991; 10:491-498.

48. Baldwin JC, Wolfgang TC, Shumway NE, Lower RR. Cardiac transplantation. In: Flye MW, ed, Principles of Organ Transplantation. Philadelphia, PA: WB Saunders, 1989:385-402.

49. Evans RW. Financial aspects of organ transplantation: A summary of the results from the national cooperative transplantation study. In: Evans RW, Manninen DL, Dong FB, eds. The National Cooperative Transplantation Study: Final Report. Seattle: Battelle-Seattle Research Center, June 1991.

50. Evans RW. Executive Summary: The National Cooperative Transplantation Study. Report BHARC-100-91-020. Seattle, WA Battelle-Seattle Research Center, June 1991.

51. Kjellstrand CM. Age, sex, and race inequality in renal transplantation. Arch Intern Med 1988; 148:135-139.

52. Hagle ME, Rosenberg JC, Lysz K, Kaplan MP, Sillix D, Jr. Racial perspectives on kidney transplant donors and recipients. Transplantation 1989; 48:421-424.

53. Office of Inspector General. Office of Evaluations and Inspections. The distribution of organs for transplantation: Expectations and practices. Washington, DC: Government Printing Office, 1990. (DHHS publication no. (OEI) 01-89-00550).

54. Evans RW. Public and private insurer designation of transplantation programs. Transplantation, in press.

55. Renlund DG, Bristow MR, Lybert MR, O'Connell JB, Gay WA, Jr. Medicare-designated centers for cardiac transplantation. N Engl J Med 1987; 316:873-876.

56. Evans RW. Medicare-designated centers for cardiac transplantation (letter). N Engl J Med 1987; 317:966.

57. Health Insurance Association of America. Organ transplants and their implications for the health insurance industry. Washington, DC Health Insurance Association of America; 1985.

58. Koska MT. Institutes of quality experience uneven volume. Hospitals. 1990; 64(3):44,46-48.

59. Evans RW, Dong FB, Manninen DL. The center effect in heart transplantation. In: Evans RW, Manninen DL, Dong FB, eds. The National Cooperative Transplantation Study: Final report. Seattle: Battelle-Seattle Research Center, June 1991.

60. Evans RW. The center effect in transplantation. In: Evans RW, Manninen DL, Dong FB, eds. The National Cooperative Transplantation Study: Final report. Seattle: Battelle-Seattle Research Center, June 1991.

61. The Working Group on Mechanical Circulatory Support of the National Heart, Lung, and Blood Institute. Artificial heart and assist devices: Directions, needs, costs, societal and ethical issues. Bethesda: National Heart, Lung and Blood Institute, 1985.

62. Culliton BJ. Politics of the heart. Science 1988; 241:283.

63. Booth W. A change of heart. Science 1988; 240:976.

64. Pierce WS. Permanent heart substitution: Better solutions lie ahead. JAMA 1988; 259:891.

65. Pae WE, Jr, Pierce WS. Combined registry for the clinical use of mechanical ventricular assist pumps and the total artificial heart: Second official report—1987. J Heart Transplantation 1989; 8:1-4.

66. Goldsmith MF. Fully implanted life ventricular assist device may enter clinical trials early in 1991. JAMA 1990; 263:2990-2991.

67. Goldsmith MF. First implant of portable heart-assist device. JAMA 1991; 265:2930-2933.

68. Caplan AL. Ethical issues raised by research involving xenografts. JAMA 1985; 254:3339-3343.

69. Council on Scientific Affairs Xenografts: Review of the literature and current status. JAMA 1985; 254:3353-3357.

70. Sadeghi AM, Laks H, Drinkwater DC et al. Heart-lung xenotransplantation in primates. J Heart Lung Transplant 1991; 10:442-448.

71. Evans RW. Failure despite success: An impartial perspective on the current status of organ transplantation procedures and policy. In: Evans RW, Manninen DL, Dong FB, eds. The National Cooperative Transplantation Study: Final report. Seattle: Battelle-Seattle Research Center, June 1991.

===================== CHAPTER 2 =====================

HEART DONOR MANAGEMENT

D.K.C. Cooper

INTRODUCTION

Worldwide, the one-year survival after heart transplantation is approximately 80%. The Registry of the International Society for Heart and Lung Transplantation reports that 25% of the deaths are directly related to donor heart failure, which, therefore, accounts for 5% of the overall mortality in the first year. As approximately 2,500 heart transplants are performed worldwide annually, approximately 125 patients die in the early hours or days after transplantation because the donor heart does not function adequately. This is clearly an area, therefore, where considerable improvement can be made in the overall results of transplantation.

It is my belief, from more than 13 years experience in the field of clinical heart transplantation, that many of these deaths from donor heart failure can be avoided by improved selection and management of donors, even given the limited knowledge we have today of the events that take place in the body after brain death.

In the last consecutive 100 patients who underwent heart transplantation at our own center in Oklahoma City, we have documented only one death related to donor heart failure, and this was in an exceptional circumstance where the aircraft bringing the donor heart from a distant center was diverted because of adverse weather conditions to another state. The overall ischemic period was almost seven hours, and the heart initially failed to function adequately. Although it subsequently recovered after a period supported by a ventricular assist device, the patient suffered a major cerebrovascular accident, from which he did not recover.

With this exception, however, donor function has been adequate, and usually good, though some inotropic support has been almost universally administered for the first 24 to 48 hours. For a period of time, it was our policy to give hormonal therapy to the donor in the form of triiodothyronine (T3) (see below), but for the past 12 months or so we have not done so and have seen no deterioration in our functional results. This has reassured us that, with careful selection and management based on well-accepted hemodynamic principles, the majority of donor hearts will function satisfactorily after transplantation if the ischemic interval is less than approximately four hours.

However, there remain a small number of donors who are hemodynamically unstable and who, despite adequate management, may continue so. Careful assessment of such donors is therefore essential before a decision is made to use the heart for transplantation. Our own policy in this respect in recent years has been one of conservatism. If we have had serious doubts about donor heart viability, then we have erred on the side of caution. The decision may at times be extremely difficult and is largely based on previous experience. It is therefore important that the surgeon who assesses the donor and removes the heart should have significant experience in this regard.

It is to this group of unstable or inadequate donors that we must concentrate our attention. If we can find methods to "stabilize" them, the same methods may also improve the function of the stable donors.

How can we improve the management of such donors in the hope that more of them will be "salvaged" and thus become suitable for purposes of transplantation? In other words, can we "resuscitate" poorly functioning hearts whilst they remain in the donor (or at the time of cardioplegic arrest and/or during the period of ex vivo preservation) to enable them to become acceptable for transplantation?

To be able to resuscitate poorly functioning donor hearts, we need to know far more about the pathophysiology associated with brain death and the metabolic and physiologic changes that take place in the donor after brain death has occurred. Despite some studies in this field, it remains a very under-investigated subject, and could be a most rewarding area for laboratory and clinical research during the next decade.

WHAT DO WE KNOW ABOUT THE EFFECTS OF BRAIN DEATH?

Experimental work in the early 80s by the Cape Town group in South Africa (Novitzky and his colleagues) documented two major findings.

The first was that myocardial injury can occur during the development of brain death (during the period of raised intracranial pressure), and is related to endogenous catecholamine release in the myocardium, which, in turn, is secondary to massive sympathetic nervous stimulation. The histopathological

nature of this injury consists of contraction bands, focal coagulative necrosis, and myocytolysis, with edema formation and interstitial mononuclear cell infiltration. Contraction band necrosis may even develop in conduction tissue and coronary arterial smooth muscle.

Although the injury can be reduced to some degree by prior therapy with beta adrenergic blockers or calcium antagonists (or total cardiac sympathectomy), this is clearly rarely possible in the clinical situation. The donor may already have undergone these pathophysiologic changes, often acutely, before he enters the hospital and certainly before he is first seen by the cardiac transplant surgeon. These changes cannot, therefore, be prevented under clinical conditions, and we have to accept that a certain number of hearts will have suffered some injury before the patient is considered as a donor.

The second significant finding in the brain-dead donor related to certain metabolic changes that were documented in the experimental animal and, to a lesser degree, in the human potential donor. Significant depletion of certain plasma hormones occurs, particularly of triiodothyronine (T3), resulting in inhibition of mitochondrial function, leading to reduced aerobic metabolic oxidative processes (with increased anaerobic metabolism), affecting the body as a whole. Major organ energy stores (including those of the heart) are diminished, leading to deterioration of function and eventual cardiac arrest.

These findings correlate well with previous clinical observations that document the fact that, even if the brain-dead subject is given full intensive support (ventilation, correction of acid-base balance, inotropes, etc.), myocardial function deteriorates and cardiac arrest occurs in the majority of cases within 48-72 hours.

DONOR PRETREATMENT (HORMONAL THERAPY) - IS IT BENEFICIAL?

Having documented the above changes, the Cape Town group went on to suggest that it might be possible to maintain or improve donor heart function by taking steps to normalize the metabolism of the donor. For example, the administration of (depleted) hormones might prove beneficial.

This has been done under both experimental and clinical conditions, and the results of these studies have been published. The findings were that in the experimental animal the administration of T3 had a beneficial effect in that it led to a return to aerobic metabolism, with replacement of essential myocardial energy stores, with an associated improvement in hemodynamic performance. In the clinical arena, there was also evidence that therapy resulted in reduced anaerobic metabolism and improved cardiac function. None of these clinical studies, however, were randomized trials, and none of them were carried out by surgeons or physicians who were unaware of the therapy they were giving —in other words, they were not "blinded" studies. This work, therefore, remains controversial, and has never adequately been confirmed by other groups. In particular, the important role of T3 therapy remains unsubstantiated in a well-controlled trial.

Clinical studies from Osaka in Japan (Yoshioka and colleagues) have demonstrated that a brain-dead patient can be maintained in an adequate hemodynamic state for many days—up to 54 days in one case—by the combined intravenous infusion of epinephrine and synethetic arginine vasopressin (ADH). Long-term support of the donor was not successful when epinephrine ($\pm$ dopamine) was administered alone, even in large doses.

If the Cape Town thesis that donor myocardial energy stores become depleted after brain death is correct, then these Japanese observations suggest that the combination of epinephrine and vasopressin maintains or replaces these stores. However, measurements of the myocardial energy stores (and the state of aerobic/anaerobic metabolism) were not made in these potential donors, and so the exact reasons for the effectiveness of this therapy remain uncertain. Nevertheless, although the quality of function of organs such as the liver and kidneys was not documented, the heart clearly maintained an adequate blood pressure and cardiac output and, therefore, would seem likely to have been metabolically normal in an adequate aerobic milieu. Subsequent studies from Japan have suggested that liver stores are also satisfactorily preserved in brain-dead donors maintained on epinephrine and vasopressin.

It has been pointed out that these observations suggest that the concept that brain death leads inevitably to somatic death may be exaggerated. The fact that some brain-dead patients demonstrate longer spontaneous bodily survival than others may be related to intact posterior pituitary function (with continuing secretion of vasopressin).

This subject of hormonal depletion and therapeutic replacement is therefore clearly one where further well-controlled experimental and clinical research is required. The metabolic changes that take place in the body as a whole, and in the heart in particular, need clarification by further detailed studies. Only then will we be able to plan scientifically to improve myocardial function in the donor.

Other—quite different—forms of therapy should also be explored. For example, it is well-known that a long period of cold ischemia of the heart results in impaired function. The Cape Town group showed clearly that this impairment is significantly greater if the heart is excised from an animal that has been subjected to the pathophysiologic and metabolic changes associated with brain death. These changes almost certainly result in a relative ischemia of certain tissues and/or organs, including the heart. This has been documented both by EKG changes (transient or persistent) and histopathology. This ischemic injury may be exaggerated by the periods of cold ischemia (during transportation) and relatively warm ischemia (during insertion into the recipient) to which the heart is subsequently subjected. After transplantation, therefore, reperfusion of an organ from a brain-dead donor may lead to an increased production of oxygen free radicals (compared to that which occurs after reperfusion of an organ from a living subject). Therapy to the recipient—or even to the donor—with oxygen free radical scavengers (even when the ischemic period has been brief) may therefore prove particularly beneficial.

I believe that during the next few years

we shall see further studies of the brain-dead donor, and that these will lead to successful pretreatment to maintain not only the heart, but all of the other organs, in perfect condition for purposes of transplantation. It should then prove possible to maintain a donor in a metabolically and hemodynamically stable state for many hours or even several days. Although this latter period is unlikely to become the clinical norm (in view of the donor family's frequent request that organ excision be carried out as soon as possible so that funeral arrangements can proceed), stability of the donor would allow excision of organs to be carried out electively rather than as a semi-emergency, which would be advantageous in several respects.

"RESUSCITATION" BY IMPROVED CARDIOPLEGIC SOLUTIONS

There is a further field where major improvements could still take place, and this is in the constitution of the solution used to induce cardiac arrest and/or to store the heart during the ischemic period. The currently available commercial solutions, such as St. Thomas's Hospital solution (Plegisol), are generally adequate in preserving reasonable function if the donor heart is in a good condition before excision and if the ischemic period is not prolonged.

Even so, the Papworth group in Cambridge in the U.K. (Cankovic-Darracott and her colleagues) has clearly documented that, although approximately half of "good" donor hearts continue to show satisfactory function after transplantation, the remainder show a significant deterioration during the ischemic period and perform poorly in the recipient. Biopsies of muscle fibers from both groups of hearts demonstrate a good response to adenosine triphosphate and calcium (as measured by quantitative birefringence) prior to excision, but a marked deterioration in the post-transplant response is observed in half of the hearts. There is a higher overall mortality in these patients with impaired donor hearts, even though this mortality is sometimes related to distant factors such as acute rejection (possibly associated with increased HLA anti-

gen expression on the surface of an "injured" organ).

This work has shown that, even though the heart may appear perfectly satisfactory in the donor, a period of ischemic arrest can lead to significant deterioration in heart function (which could not be anticipated). As this deterioration does not occur in every case and is not related solely to the length of the ischemic period, it is almost certainly the result of a combination of myocardial injuries, with that associated with the effects of brain death playing a major role.

Donor heart pretreatment before excision may be the answer to this problem, but there is clearly room for improvement in the nature of the cardioplegic agent that we employ. Work by Wicomb and Collins in San Francisco in the U.S.A. has shown that improved cardioplegic agents result in significantly less deterioration of cardiac function. For example, if a rabbit heart is arrested using St. Thomas's Hospital solution at 4°C, immediate in vitro testing demonstrates a cardiac output that is approximately only 50% compared with that obtained following arrest with a recently-developed solution from Wicomb's laboratory (Cardiosol), which includes polyethylene glycol 20M as a major constituent. For many years, therefore, we would seem to have been using cardioplegic agents that are significantly less than optimal.

If the functional deterioration that results from inadequate myocardial protection is added to that which may have already occurred during brain death or during the subsequent few hours before heart excision, then it can easily be understood why donor heart function after transplantation is sometimes poor. Indeed, it is perhaps surprising that function is at least adequate in the majority of cases!

The added effect of brain death in combination with storage of the heart has already been alluded to. In the Cape Town study, hearts taken from anesthetized pigs and subsequently stored for 24 hours by continuous hypothermic perfusion showed a minimal reduction in subsequent myocardial function and no reduction in myocardial high-energy phosphates. However, if the heart was taken from a brain-dead animal (that had been hemodynamically supported by intravenous fluids, dobutamine, and/or vasopressin), subsequent function was shown to be significantly reduced. Similarly, this function was worse than that of a pig heart tested immediately after brain death (but not stored).

New solutions or modifications to existing solutions therefore offer us a real hope of improved post-transplant cardiac function in the future. Although this topic may best be discussed under the heading of "preservation of the heart," it can equally be considered as part of donor heart management as it involves, at the very least, the maintenance of donor heart function as it existed before excision. It is only one further step to develop a cardioplegic or other agent that might actually *improve* (rather than just maintain) donor heart function, and I do not believe that this is beyond the realms of possibility within the next few years.

Ideally, therefore, in 10 years time we may find ourselves in the enviable position where we are able not only to correct donor heart metabolism, increase myocardial energy stores, and improve cardiac function whilst the heart remains in the donor, but we might also be able to improve it further at the time of administration of the cardioplegic agent, and then maintain that improved status throughout a prolonged period of ischemic arrest. Immediate cardiac function in the recipient would therefore be at an optimal level, and the early progress of the patient would be greatly enhanced. As there may well be a relationship between ischemic injury to the myocardium and the development of acute rejection, the prognosis would be improved further.

VIABILITY ASSESSMENT OF THE DONOR HEART

An important aspect of our plan to obtain highly viable and immediately functional donor hearts is our need to be able to measure (before excision) the subsequent "viability" of the heart. At the present time, as outlined earlier, assessment of the viability of the organ and its anticipated future function are determined by the cardiac donor surgical team.

This team may or may not be experienced and their (subjective) assessment may or may not be accurate. Unfortunately, there is no single objective measurement or group of measurements that clearly predict which hearts will function satisfactorily after transplantation and which will not.

Several attempts have been made in the past to develop some form of viability assay or functional assessment of the donor heart. These have included histochemical staining of myocardial biopsies and functional assessment by a combination of hemodynamic measurements. None of these has to-date proved totally reliable.

Ideally, such a viability assay or functional assessment should be based on one simple measurement, whether it be by biopsy (such as that used by the Papworth group) or functional measurement. The result of the test must be available almost immediately in order that the transplant surgeon can know the viability of the organ at any single moment.

All of the studies performed by the Papworth group have been retrospective—that is, although the biopsies have been taken at various time intervals during the care of the donor and recipient, the assays have not been carried out until a later date. The test, however, would appear to be suitable to be performed at the donor center and for the result to be available in a relatively short period of time (approximately 30 minutes). However, as described above, this test does not actually *predict* donor heart function after transplantation. It can detect those hearts that are already in a poor state of viability and differentiate these from those that remain in a good state, but it cannot identify those "good" hearts that will deteriorate during transportation. A more sensitive test that can do this is therefore urgently required.

At our own center in Oklahoma City, Yokoyama and his colleagues have recently employed a catheter which measures the left ventricular end-systolic pressure-volume relationship, and we have some pilot studies that suggest that such measurements may confirm donor heart functional status. In 13 donors where both clinical parameters and pressure-volume relationship appeared to be good, all hearts were transplanted and all functioned satisfactorily. In two hearts, where we had significant clinical doubts about the donor heart status, these were confirmed by poor pressure-volume measurements; we elected not to use these hearts for transplantation.

This small initial study clearly does not answer the question fully, for we did not transplant the two hearts of which we had doubts, and therefore remain uncertain as to their subsequent function. However, previous work carried out in Japan using the same catheter in the experimental animal has demonstrated that the results obtained with it correlate closely with subsequent cardiac function.

There is undoubtedly room for much further research in this area. The development of a simple, reproducible and rapid viability test or functional assessment would be invaluable, and it is hoped that increasing attention will be paid to this potentially rewarding field in the next few years. It would seem that a test based on biopsy would be preferable to one based on functional measurement. Myocardial biopsies could be taken at intervals throughout the transplantation procedure—when the donor is first seen, after donor pretreatment, after varying periods of cold ischemic storage, etc.—ensuring that the viability status of the donor heart is known at all times. The transplant operation could thus be cancelled if the donor heart status was deteriorating significantly. It would be much more difficult—if not impossible—to carry out functional monitoring in the same way. Nevertheless, a functional measurement that confirmed good function before excision would be valuable and would at least be a first step towards ensuring that inadequate hearts were not transplanted.

We may ultimately find, therefore, that not only can we improve heart function in the donor, and further improve and/or maintain it at the time of cardioplegic arrest and storage, but that we can also confirm donor heart viability status throughout the transplantation process by a simple myocardial biopsy assay. The mortality and morbidity associated with an inadequate donor heart would then be minimized or, at best, excluded completely.

WILL WE BE ABLE TO RESUSCITATE AND UTILIZE "DEAD" HEARTS?

This is surely the final question we must ask ourselves. Will we ever be able to use the heart that has already arrested—for example, from exsanguination or anoxia? If so, what will be the maximum period of arrest compatible with successful resuscitation?

The number of donors (of all organs) available to us would be considerably increased if we could develop a technique to resuscitate such arrested hearts. With the critical shortage of suitable donors at the present time, the need for such a technique is urgent, but little research has been directed towards this problem.

Under ideal conditions, an arrested heart can certainly be excised, transplanted, and function well. Indeed, this was the case in the first heart allotransplant ever performed by Barnard and his team. The donor was taken to the operating room and prepared for surgery. Ventilation was then discontinued and the surgical team (and medical examiner) watched and waited until the heart stopped beating and the patient could be certified dead (documented by an absence of spontaneous respiratory movements, reflexes, and coordinated EKG for 5 minutes). A median sternotomy was then performed and the donor rapidly placed on cardiopulmonary bypass. Total body cooling to $26°C$ was carried out, and then the heart was selectively cooled a further $10°$ (to $16°C$).

Perfusion was discontinued and the heart excised and carried to the adjoining operating room where the recipient had already been placed on pump-oxygenator support. Whilst the donor heart was being inserted, the myocardium was protected by coronary perfusion using cooled recipient blood from the pump-oxygenator. Immediate post-transplant function was excellent.

What we are considering now, however, is rather different. We would hope to utilize a heart that is perhaps rapidly failing in the emergency room (or has already ceased functioning by the time the patient reaches the emergency room). The technique we would require would almost certainly necessitate immediate and rapid cannulation of the femoral artery and vein, initiation of total body cooling by a pump-oxygenator, transfer of the patient to the operating room, and excision of organs.

Although not totally unfeasible, there are a number of practical problems associated with this concept. A pump-oxygenator facility (machine and, possibly, technician also) would need to be available in the emergency room at all times. Although next-of-kin consent might not be required to initiate cardiopulmonary bypass (though this is a moot legal point as cardiopulmonary bypass is being initiated not to preserve the life of the patient but only to preserve him as a potential organ donor), the relatives would need to be contacted as soon as possible to provide consent for organ donation.

It is even possible, of course, that the patient might recover fully or partially—some cerebral function, for example. How would the patient then be managed? He would no longer be a candidate for donation and yet might be dependent on pump-oxygenator support. An accurate determination of cerebral function would not be possible if the body temperature had been reduced to a low level, yet myocardial protection might be jeopardized if the patient were rewarmed to normothermia.

The concept is, therefore, fraught with practical problems, and much time and effort to "salvage" donors in this way might go unrewarded. Nevertheless, under certain conditions, it might prove feasible. In the patient who is certified dead in the emergency room— no heart beat, flat EKG, fixed dilated pupils, thrombosis of the retinal vessels, etc—the rapid employment of hypothermic cardiopulmonary bypass using the femoral vessels might provide an opportunity for adequate "resuscitation" of the heart (and other organs).

Personal laboratory studies carried out over 20 years ago demonstrated that canine hearts that had arrested following exsanguination could be resuscitated to some considerable degree if the warm ischemic period did not extend beyond 60 minutes. If the arrest resulted from asphyxia (anoxia), which appeared more damaging to the myocardium, then resuscitation was less successful but could still be achieved if the ischemic period were relatively short (less than approximately 30 minutes).

Resuscitation in these experiments was not by the use of cardiopulmonary bypass, but was achieved by isolating the heart and lungs from the rest of the body (by clamping the SVC, IVC and aorta) followed by the institution of ventilation and manual cardiac massage (±infusion of blood). The circulation induced by massage was limited to the coronary and pulmonary circulations, thus reducing the workload placed on the myocardium and isolating the heart from the (toxic) effects of ischemia in other organs, such as the liver. After relatively short periods of massage, oxygenation, and correction of acid-base balance, electrical defibrillation was attempted with success in many cases.

It would seem, therefore, that the heart may tolerate a short period of warm ischemic arrest and that severe, irreversible injury is not inevitable. If we can develop methods that allow the heart to recover from the warm ischemic injury, then we may be able to use some hearts that are presently not available to us as donor organs. This is yet another area that has been inadequately investigated and is worthy of study.

COMMENT

Donor heart management has possibly been perceived as one of the less rewarding and less "glamorous" aspects of heart transplantation. We need to impress upon our young research colleagues that it is an essential and important field of transplantation to which they could profitably apply their attention and research endeavors. If successful, the results of their labors would have an immediate impact on clinical heart transplantation.

As this volume is dedicated to the future, however, it has to be pointed out that all aspects of management of the brain-dead organ donor may rapidly pass into the realm of medical history once the problems inherent in xenotransplantation have been overcome— which may not be too far in the future.

CHAPTER 3

SELECTION AND MANAGEMENT OF THE LUNG DONOR

Thomas M. Egan

INTRODUCTION

The major impediment to more widespread application of lung transplantation is the lack of suitable pulmonary donors. This chapter will focus on criteria for suitable pulmonary donors, discuss optimal management of the pulmonary donor, and explore methods that may improve the donor pool.

CURRENT TRANSPLANT DONOR POOL

Few studies have addressed the issue of the potential number of organ donors in the United States. Bart et al, from the Center for Disease Control, analyzed 12,531 in-hospital deaths and estimated a prevalence of 59 potential organ donors/million population/year.[1] This would translate to more than 15,000 donors across the United States and substantiates approximations that only 10 to 20% of potential organ donors actually come to any form of organ retrieval. In one study of fatal head injuries, denial of consent of next of kin accounted for 34% of failures to retrieve organs from potential donors, implying that lack of acceptance of the concept of organ donation is a major problem.[2] Failure to request on the part of the medical personnel caring for the donor was identified in 30% of potential donors in a pool of nontrauma patients.[3]

The subset of donors with lungs that are suitable for transplantation is smaller still, for a number of reasons. Brain death mandates intubation and mechanical ventilation, bypassing the upper respiratory airway defense mechanisms. This results in colonization of the airway and predisposes to pneumonia. Aspiration is frequently associated with trauma or other events preceding brain death. Chest trauma is a frequent accompaniment of closed head injury, which may preclude suitable lung function if pulmonary contusion occurs. Neurogenic pulmonary edema is another cause of pulmonary dysfunction in brain-injured patients. The mechanism for this is poorly understood but is believed related to "catecholamine storm" and, experimentally, can be related to poor cardiac function.[4] Nevertheless, in a recent study of cardiac donors, it was estimated that perhaps as many as 25% of cardiac donors may have lungs suitable for transplantation.[5] Despite this, there were 262 isolated lung transplants and 50 heart/lung transplants performed in the United States in 1990, compared with 2,085 heart transplants,[6] so it would appear that there are potentially more pulmonary donors that are not being utilized at present. This situation may be resolved with improved awareness and strategies adopted by UNOS to improve pulmonary retrieval.

CHARACTERISTICS OF A PULMONARY DONOR

Ideally, all multiple organ donors should be evaluated as potential pulmonary donors for transplantation. The widely accepted published criteria[7] are listed in Table 1. A clear chest x-ray is no longer considered an absolute requirement by most experienced centers, since interstitial fluid accumulation is frequently seen, and occasionally, lungs which have been contused are suitable for transplantation. Additionally, plate atelectasis may reverse with more appropriate ventilatory parameters, and chest x-ray should be repeated with the potential donor ventilated with an adequate tidal volume (10 to 15 cc/kg) and 5 cm of PEEP. Assessment of the airway for evidence of aspiration and/or purulent tracheobronchitis

Table 1. Lung Donor Criteria[7]

Age < 55 years
Normal chest x-ray
PaO_2 300mm Hg on FiO_2 1.0, PEEP 5cm for 5 minutes
Bronchoscopically clear with no evidence of purulent secretions or aspiration
No significant chest trauma or pulmonary contusion
No previous thoracic surgery on side of harvest

is of paramount importance, but a positive gram stain of tracheal aspirate does not necessarily preclude lung donation. Both Stanford University[8] and the University of Pittsburgh[9] have reported that the incidence of tracheal colonization by gram stain in their heart-lung or lung donors was approximately 80%.

An aggressive approach to lung salvage has recently been reported by the Toronto Lung Transplant Group, in circumstances where chest radiograph or bronchoscopy documented unilateral pulmonary pathology. At organ retrieval, selective occlusion of each pulmonary artery and single lung ventilation through a Carlens tube documented gas exchange function of *each* lung. When unilateral dysfunction was documented, the lung exhibiting good gas exchange was retrieved and successfully transplanted on four occasions.[10] The quality of the secretions is a more important determinant of subsequent outcome. (Fig. 1)

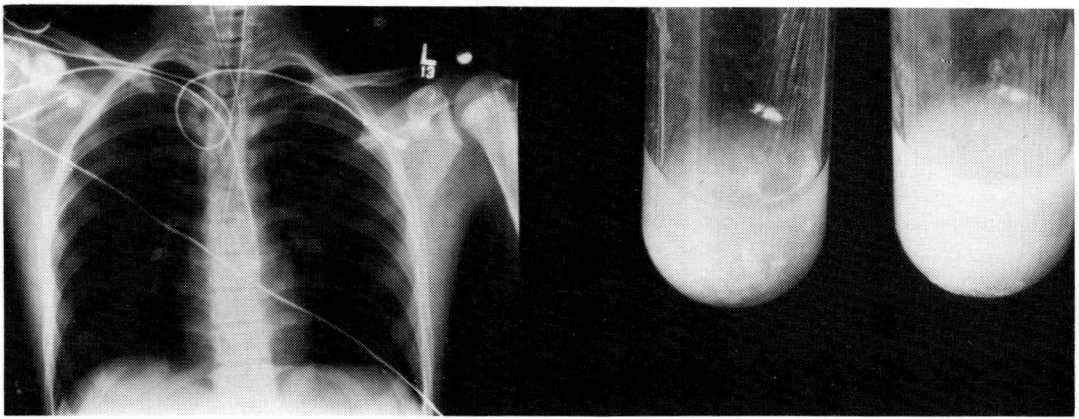

Fig. 1. Despite a clear chest x-ray (left) and excellent gas exchange, this donor had grossly purulent bronchial washings (right).

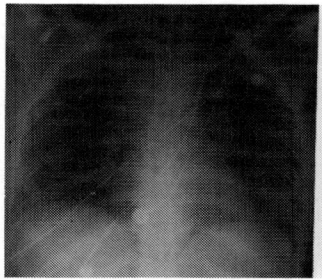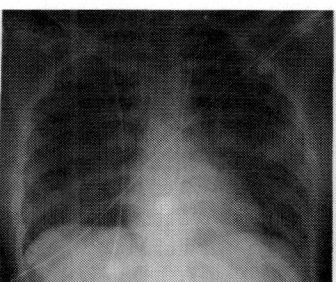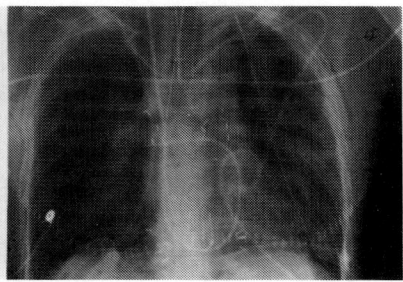

Fig. 2. Clear chest x-ray (left) of a donor with a closed head injury. Prior to organ retrieval, oxygenation deteriorated, and pulmonary edema became apparent (middle). After transplanting both lungs into a recipient with cystic fibrosis, lung fields cleared radiographically (right). The recipient had an uneventful recovery.

MANAGEMENT OF PULMONARY ORGAN DONORS

The treatment of multiple organ donors encompasses all aspects of intensive care therapy for the brain-injured patient and requires a thorough understanding of cardiopulmonary physiology and related hemodynamics. Cardiac and pulmonary dysfunction often accompanies brain injury.[4] Brain stem herniation frequently results in vasomotor instability, resulting in significant alterations in systemic vascular resistance. Diabetes insipidus occurs often after brain death, which makes intravenous fluid management difficult.[11]

In the presence of diabetes insipidus, volume requirements may be substantial to maintain perfusion pressure; however, excessive crystalloid infusion can lead to pulmonary edema and electrolyte abnormalities. While this may clear in a lung recipient *after* transplantation, most centers would be reluctant to transplant a lung with impaired gas exchange. Figure 2 depicts a sequence of radiographic changes in a lung donor who developed pulmonary edema prior to organ retrieval. Transplantation resulted in rapid clearance of the radiographic picture.

To avoid excessive volume loss and electrolyte disturbances, pitressin (0.5 to 1.0 U/hr) or desmopressin (DDAVP) 0.5 to 2.0 μg every 8-12 hours can be used to keep urine output below 250 ml/hr.[11] Low dose dopamine will often effectively counter some of the vasodilatation associated with brain stem dysfunction and may facilitate maintenance of acceptable pressure without massive fluid infusion. The use of low dose inotropes and vasopressin is preferred to "drowning" a potential lung donor with crystalloid.

The duration of ventilation prior to organ retrieval predisposes to atelectasis and increases the risk of airway contamination. Consequently, it is unusual to have acceptable gas exchange in donors ventilated beyond a week, but the duration of ventilation in and of itself is not a contraindication to pulmonary retrieval for transplantation. Because of the mandatory positive pressure ventilation, chest physiotherapy and measures to prevent atelectasis (posturing, frequent change in position) are important aspects of the management of these patients. Frequently, the management of the brain injury that precedes brain death includes no PEEP and low tidal volume/high respiratory rate ventilation. Once brain death has been established, more aggressive ventilatory management is preferable, and assessment of gas exchange can be realistically performed only in the setting of adequate tidal volume (15 cc/kg) with the presence of physiologic amounts of PEEP.

Experimental brain death is associated with depletion of circulating thyroxine, cortisol, and insulin.[4] Based on animal data that hormonal therapy could improve myocardial energy stores and function after transplantation,[12] brain dead potential organ donors have been treated with these hormones, with encouraging effects on hemodynamics.[13] If this approach renders donors more hemodynamically stable, then it may increase salvage of lungs by reducing pulmonary edema.

CRITERIA FOR DONOR SELECTION

Aside from adequate pulmonary function and a lack of infection in the donor, there are certain recipient characteristics that require consideration. As for all solid organs, ABO compatibility is a requisite for successful transplantation. With ABO compatible but not identical transplantation, there is a risk of transient hemolytic anemia, which is usually well tolerated.

The present state of the art for lung preservation precludes HLA matching among lung or heart-lung donors and recipients. While there appeared to be an advantage to HLA matching for renal grafts in the pre-cyclosporine era,[14] this issue has not been addressed in the lung.

Some centers have advocated "CMV matching"—that is, avoiding transplantation of lungs from a CMV positive donor into a CMV negative recipient, because of the severity of the subsequent CMV pneumonitis in the immunocompromised host.[15] Since the introduction of ganciclovir for successful therapy of CMV disease in lung recipients,[16] most programs do not require CMV matching, although it may reduce the severity of disease.

Size matching is of considerable importance. A lung too large for the pleural space in which it is placed will be subject to atelectasis in the recipient, and clearance of secretions in the early postoperative period will be impaired. In general, the appropriate sized transplant is the ideal size of the lung for the recipient if the recipient did not have lung disease.[17] Because total lung capacity is a function of height, age, and sex, the heights of the recipient and donor are more appropriate indicators for size matching than are their respective weights.

Recipients with obstructive lung disease have hyperexpanded chests that will accommodate a lung with a size larger than predicted. After transplant, the chest will remodel to some extent, both in terms of diaphragmatic contour and overall circumference. Conversely, patients with restrictive lung disease have a chest cavity that has often been reduced in size by the fibrotic process involving the lung parenchyma. Fortunately, placing a larger lung in this chest usually results in a mediastinal shift to the opposite hemithorax and accommodation of an appropriate sized lung. Once again, one can anticipate that in usual circumstances, the chest will increase in size over several months following transplantation. Placing too small a lung into a pleural space runs the risk of pleural space problems, but also will likely afford too small a vascular surface area. "Hyperexpansion" of a small lung is likely detrimental and may induce a significant pulmonary injury. Larger donor lungs may adapt to a small recipient chest cavity.[18] Larger lungs can also be "downsized" by a variety of methods including lobectomy or non-anatomic size reduction using stapling apparatus. On three occasions we have performed right middle lobectomy to allow a double lung block to be accommodated into the chest of a recipient, and in one instance we also performed partial lingulectomy using a stapling device because of a donor/recipient size mismatch.

FUTURE DIRECTIONS

Various strategies have been proposed to increase the number of organ donors in general, which would ultimately increase the number of lung donors. Financial incentives to donor families have been debated, but there are ethical and moral concerns.[19] Improved mechanisms for organ distribution should identify more pulmonary donors among the current pool of cadaveric organ donors. It is reasonable to anticipate that in most instances, a lung block can be used for transplant in a double lung recipient or two single lung recipients. Relaxation of current criteria for pulmonary donors will likely result as more experience is gained by transplant centers, particularly with reference to reversibility of neurogenic pulmonary edema and fluid overload in donors.

Experience with lobe transplants from parents to offspring has been very limited.*

---

*V. Starnes, Stanford University, personal communication; and R. Bolman, University of Minnestoa, personal communication.

This may become particularly useful for pediatric patients, since the number of conventional pediatric donors is likely lower than the number of potential pediatric lung recipients. It is not clear how much pulmonary tissue is required for safe transplantation when one is considering a lobe transplant into a child, nor is it clear whether this lobe will grow with the child. Nevertheless, the prospect of living related donors may afford an exciting opportunity to provide pulmonary tissue for needy recipients in the pediatric age group.

Some animal data are available that would support consideration of true cadavers as lung donors. The lung is unique among solid organs in that it does not rely on perfusion for the cellular function of respiration. Respiration occurs in the lung across a gas phase and, accordingly, the lung likely remains viable for a period of time after cessation of circulation. Lungs retrieved one hour after death provide excellent gas exchange function following transplantation in a non-survival dog model.[20] Ventilation of the cadaver donor improves outcome of transplantation of lungs retrieved four hours after death.[21] A more thorough understanding of the time course of irreversible pulmonary parenchymal ischemic damage will allow for broader application of this concept.

Ultimately, xenografting will provide a solution to the shortage of suitable lungs for transplantation, but this next chapter in lung transplantation awaits further developments in immunology.

SUMMARY

The number of suitable lung donors among the current pool of multiple organ donors in the United States is insufficient to meet the growing demand for organs among recipients. Aspiration and airway infection provide major obstacles to successful lung transplantation. Performing single lung transplant when feasible will allow for larger numbers of recipients to undergo lung transplantation. Careful fluid management of donors with judicious use of inotropes and vasopressin may optimize the number of lung donors in the current pool. Future prospects for increasing the donor pool include the use of living related donors for pediatric transplant, potentially the use of circulation arrested cadavers as lung donors, and ultimately the use of xenografts.

REFERENCES

1. Bart KJ, Macon EJ, Humphries AL et al. Increasing the supply of cadaveric kidneys for transplantation. Transplantation 1981; 31:383-387.
2. Mackersie RC, Bronsther OL, Shackford SR. Organ procurement in patients with fatal head injuries: The fate of the potential donor. Ann Surg 1991; 213:143-150.
3. Morris JA Jr, Wilcox TR, Noreuil T, Frist WH. Organ donation: A university hospital experience. South Med J 1990; 83:884-888.
4. Novitsky D, Wicomb WN, Cooper DKC et al. Electrocardiographic, hemodynamic, and endocrine changes occurring during experimental brain death in the chacma baboon. J Heart Transplant 1984; 4:63-69.
5. Egan TM, Boychuk J, Rosato CR, Cooper JD. Whence the lungs? A study to assess suitability of donor lungs for transplantation. Transplantation, in press.
6. UNOS Update 7:1-2, 1991.
7. Egan TM, Kaiser L, Cooper JD. Lung transplantation. Curr Prob Surg 1989; 26:675-751.
8. Harjula A, Starnes VA, Oyer PE et al. Proper donor selection for heart-lung transplantation: The Stanford experience. J Thorac Cardiovasc Surg 1987; 94:874-880.
9. Griffith BP, Zenati M. The pulmonary donor. Clin Chest Med 1990; 11:217-226.
10. Puskas JD, Winton TL, Miller J et al. Unilateral donor lung dysfunction does not preclude successful contralateral single lung transplantation. J Thorac Cardiovasc Surg, in press.
11. Darby JM, Stein K, Grenvik A, Stuart SA. Approach to management of the heartbeating "brain dead" organ donor. JAMA 1989; 261:2222-2228.
12. Novitzky D, Wicomb WN, Cooper DKC, Tjaalgard MA. Improved cardiac function following hormonal therapy in brain dead pigs: Relevance to organ donation. Cryobiology 1987; 24:1-10.
13. Novitzky D, Cooper DKC, Reichart B. Hemodynamic and metabolic responses to hormonal therapy in brain-dead potential organ donors. Transplantation 1987; 43:852-854.
14. Sanfilippo F, Vaughn WK, Spees EK et al. Benefits of HLA-A and HLA-B matching on graft and patient outcome after cadaveric-donor renal transplantation. New Engl J Med 1984; 311:358-364.
15. Wreghitt TG, Hakim M, Gray JJ et al. Cytomegalovirus infections in heart and heart and lung transplant recipients. J Clin Pathol 1988; 41:660-667.

16. Keay S, Petersen E, Icenogle T et al. Ganciclovir treatment of serious cytomegalovirus infection in heart and heart-lung transplant recipients. Rev Infec Dis 1988; 10(Suppl):S563-S572.

17. Miyoshi S, Schaefers H-J, Trulock EP et al. Donor selection for single and double lung transplantation: Chest size matching and other factors influencing posttransplantation vital capacity. Chest 1990; 98:308-313.

18. Lloyd KS, Barnard P, Holland VA et al. Pulmonary function after heart-lung transplantation using larger donor organs. Am Rev Respir Dis 1990; 142:1026-1029.

19. Peters PG. Life or death: The issue of payment in cadaveric organ donation. JAMA 1991; 265:1302-1305.

20. Egan TM, Lambert CJ Jr, Reddick RL et al. A strategy to increase the donor pool: The use of cadaver lungs for transplantation. Ann Thorac Surg 1991; 52:1113-21.

21. Ulicny KS Jr, Egan TM, Lambert CJ Jr et al. Immediate postmortem ventilation improves pulmonary function after transplantation. Ann Thorac Surg, in press.

CHAPTER 4

CLINICAL COMPLICATIONS OF HEART TRANSPLANTATION: PRESENT AND FUTURE TRENDS

David E. Tolman   P. K. Mohanty

Peter D. Taylor   Michael L. Hess

INTRODUCTION

Cardiac transplantation has become an accepted and important therapeutic modality for patients with end-stage congestive heart failure. Cardiac transplantation, at least initially, produces complete denervation of the heart, thus depriving the heart of important neural regulating mechanisms. Despite this, the ability of the anatomically denervated heart to support the circulatory demands of ordinary physical activity by the recipient (by atypical adoptive mechanisms) remains relatively preserved. In recent years, improved immunosuppression, largely due to cyclosporine, has significantly enhanced the long-term (5-10 years) survival following cardiac transplantation. However, hypertension, renal insufficiency, accelerated coronary arteriopathy and subsequent allograft dysfunction are emerging as major limiting factors for extended survival in cardiac transplant recipients.

This chapter will describe the state-of-the-art and future expectations for the clinical complications of heart transplantation. It is important to emphasize that the immediate postoperative surgical complications have been extensively reviewed in the past five years and these complications and their management are not expected to change dramatically. Therefore, the focus will be to discuss the major medical complications of cardiac transplantation and speculate on future trends. We will describe early postoperative complications which include (a) low cardiac output syndromes, (b) cardiac arrhythmias, and (c) cardiac allograft rejection. For the long-term post-transplant complications we will discuss post-transplant hypertension, accelerated coronary atherosclerosis, and chronic renal failure. We will then speculate and peer into the crystal ball and visualize potential future therapies of what are now well-defined problems in cardiac transplantation in the 1990s.

EARLY POST-TRANSPLANT CLINICAL COMPLICATIONS

Low Cardiac Output Syndromes

Low cardiac output is defined by a cardiac index of < 2.5 $1/min/m^2$ and occurs in heart transplant recipients for a variety of reasons including hypovolemia, myocardial injury due to prolonged ischemic time, and acute allograft rejection. Low cardiac output syndromes are easily detectable in the early post-transplant period since patients are continuously monitored by Swan-Ganz catheterization. Signs and symptoms of impaired perfusion such as hyponatremia, cool, clammy extremities, significant brady- or tachyarrhythmias, decreased urine output and elevations in creatine, BUN and liver function tests, etc. all point to a possible low cardiac output syndrome.

In a recent study[1] of early and late hemodynamic evaluation after cardiac transplantation Corcos et al demonstrated that the low output syndrome occurs in 7% of post-transplant patients. The two most serious etiologies of low cardiac output in the early post-transplant period are (a) myocardial injury due to prolonged ischemic time and (b) acute cardiac allograft rejection. The differentiation of these two conditions may present problems at the bedside and require emergent endomyocardial biopsy to rule out the presence of allograft rejection. If acute rejection is present, increased immunosuppression is necessary. However, in the absence of rejection, the etiology of low output may be "harvesting injury" and the treatment is directed toward a combination of inotropic drugs to increase cardiac output and maintain an acceptable perfusion pressure. If medical therapy does not result in adequate perfusion pressure, an intra-aortic balloon counter pulsation pump to support the systemic-circulation may become necessary. Similar therapeutic measures may on rare occasion be necessary to stabilize the hemodynamic compromise associated with acute allograft rejection until the rejection resolves and cardiac function recovers. In the rare event that both or either of these injuries are severe enough to cause irreversible damage to the myocardium resulting in the graft's inability to maintain adequate perfu-

sion pressure then replacement of the failing graft may be necessary. The total artificial heart can be used as a bridge to retransplantation and allows for improved end organ function and offers sufficient time to find a donor heart.

Other possible causes of low cardiac output include cardiac tamponade, hypovolemia, sepsis and myocardial depressant medications. The presence of a pericardial effusion, especially a posterior effusion, is readily established by two-dimensional echocardiography. An effusion leading to hemodynamic compromise is suggested by the presence of right ventricular collapse. The diagnosis of cardiac tamponade is confirmed by right heart catheterization demonstrating equalization of intracardiac pressures. Therapeutic options include percutaneous pericardiocentesis or surgical drainage and the creation of a pericardial window. The findings of low cardiac filling pressures during right heart catheterization would support the diagnosis of hypovolemia. Correction of this problem can be easily accomplished with replacement of intravascular volume and optimization of cardiac filling pressures. The major causes of hypovolemia include excessive diuresis, hemorrhage, and inadequate replacement of insensible losses. Sepsis poses a major threat to the recipient due to intense postoperative immunosuppression and the inability of the host to handle infections. Aggressive attempts at identifying the nature and site of infections with cultures of blood, urine and sputum, inspection of all suture lines, replacement of all IV and arterial catheters and a careful examination of the patient including sinuses, oral cavity, lungs, abdomen, and rectum are needed to quickly establish the diagnosis and initiate appropriate antimicrobial treatment. Concomitantly, a reduction in the level of immunosuppression may become necessary to combat and optimize life-threatening infections.

The low cardiac output syndrome may be observed during long-term follow-up and is usually related to cardiac allograft rejection, which may be either myocardial or vascular in nature. It is important to emphasize that cardiac function in the majority of patients at rest is satisfactory in both the short and long-term following cardiac transplantation.

However, mild to moderate hemodynamic abnormalities characterized by increased filling pressures (increased left ventricular end-diastolic pressure and right atrial pressures), are common in asymptomatic cardiac transplant. Of note, the transplanted heart in the absence of acute rejection has normal contractility and contractile reserve and has a normal inotropic response to beta agonists.[1]

Cardiac Arrhythmias

Recent evidence suggests that ventricular dysrhythmias occur in more than half of all cardiac transplant recipients.[1,2] A fairly high incidence of minor electrophysiological abnormalities have also been reported in completely asymptomatic patients without any evidence of rejection. These include prolonged intra-atrial conduction time thought to be secondary to surgical technique during the transplantation procedure and duality of the AV nodal conduction system.[1] In one study, atrial dysrhythmias occurred in 72% of patients and ventricular dysrhythmias in 57% of patients. In some studies dysrhythmias, especially atrial fibrillation, appear to be related to periods of acute allograft rejection.[3,1] The common causes for such rhythm disturbances include hypoxia, acidosis, hypovolemia, hypomagnesemia, acute allograft rejection or other medications including inotropic therapy. Intravenous lidocaine has been an effective drug for suppression of ventricular arrhythmias with minimal adverse effects in the transplant patient. Long-term therapy can be achieved with a variety of agents including procainamide, quinidine and tocainide.

Denervation has no protective effect on ventricular or atrial arrhythmias. Atrial dysrhythmias are more common than ventricular dysrhythmias and necessitate treatment when the ventricular response is abnormal and when the rhythm compromises the hemodynamic state of the patient. Complex premature ventricular contractions (PVCs) are: a) associated with increased mortality; b) sensitive but not specific for accelerated atherosclerosis, and c) more predictive of mortality and sudden death than simple PVCs.[4] Power spectrum analysis of heart rate variability in human cardiac transplant recipients indicates that denervation of the heart significantly reduces the normal heart rate effect variability and abolishes the discreet spectral peak seen in nontransplanted control subjects.[1] The development of allograft rejection may significantly increase the heart rate variability. Thus, power spectrum analysis may be a potential, reasonable noninvasive tool in the early diagnosis of cardiac allograft rejection.

Pharmacology of the Transplanted Heart

Data concerning the pharmacological effect of drugs on the transplanted human heart is limited and may actually change over time, if indeed reinnervation occurs. A recent study by Stark et al[8] has cast doubt on the existing premise that the transplanted heart remains permanently denervated. Stark has demonstrated that patients five or more months out from orthotopic cardiac transplantation may indeed develop limited sympathetic reinnervation. This may suggest that drugs whose effect is mediated via the autonomic nervous system (sympathetic and parasympathetic) will have little effect on the transplanted heart early on following transplantation, but over time may develop their typical pharmacodynamic profile. This possible dynamic state of denervation/reinnervation must be kept in mind when discussing the pharmacodynamic or adverse effect of any drug which is mediated via the autonomic nervous system. It is clear that following transplantation, at least in the short term, a state of denervation exists and therefore a short discussion of the side effects of this created state is in order. It must be kept in mind that these responses may change over time. A recognized side effect of denervation of the heart is "denervation hypersensitivity" which is characterized by an enhanced response to certain drugs, such as beta receptor agonists. Drugs with striking effects on the peripheral vasculature (vasodilators) and negative inotropic drugs may have a profound effect on systemic hemodynamics, since the denervated human heart relies mainly on the Starling mechanisms and cannot change contractility for a given stress response. Since digoxin, calcium antagonists, inotropic agents, antiarrhythmic agents and β blockers are commonly used following cardiac transplantation, the effects of these agents in the transplanted denervated heart will be briefly discussed.

Digoxin

The autonomic nervous system significantly modulates the effects of digoxin in normally innervated hearts, prolonging both the effective refractory period and the atrial functional refractory period, irrespective of the cycle length. However, there is a lesser effect on sinus node function, with a slight increase in sinus cycle length, sinus node recovery time and sinoatrial conduction time occurring in response to digitalis. These effects on the AV node and the sinoatrial node appear to be mediated by the autonomic nervous system. Thus in a denervated transplanted human heart, digoxin has a minimal effect on the AV node and has virtually no effect on sinus node function. The therapeutic implications of these findings are that the effects of digoxin on AV conduction is attenuated in the transplanted heart. Thus, the magnitude of slowing of the ventricular response in atrial fibrillation in patients with cardiac transplantation is significantly less than that occurring in the innervated heart. Therefore, an increased dose of digoxin may be required to produce a slowing of AV conduction.

Calcium Antagonists

The calcium antagonists, diltiazem, verapamil and nifedipine all have direct binding sites on the myocardium, and thus have a preserved effect on the denervated human heart. These drugs, however, should be used with caution since they are potential negative inotropes with significant vasodilatory properties. In addition, they also have potential interaction with cyclosporine. Therapeutic use of this concept is seen with the cyclosporine/diltiazem interaction. Diltiazem displaces cyclosporine from protein binding sites effectively increasing free serum cyclosporine levels. This allows for a lower dose of maintenance cyclosporine while concomitantly treating hypertension. A report by Schroeder et al[9] has suggested that diltiazem may also be beneficial in reducing the progression of coronary arterial narrowing in the transplanted heart following its administration. Use of nifedipine in transplant recipients has been reported to produce an exaggerated response with marked orthostatic hypotension often limiting its usefulness.

Inotropic Agents

Orthotopic cardiac transplantation with cardiac denervation results in depletion of myocardial catecholamines[1] resulting in an increased sensitivity to circulating catecholamines. Therefore, enhanced inotropic and chronotropic response to adrenaline, noradrenaline and isoprenaline can be expected in the transplanted human heart. The sensitivity appears to be mediated by a change in the state of beta adrenoreceptors. Inotropic agents such as dopamine and dobutamine, whose actions are primarily mediated by a beta adrenoreceptor, have potentially similar augmented effects[1,2] and must be titrated with caution.

Antiarrhythmic Agents

In the absence of accelerated coronary atherosclerosis, ventricular and supraventricular arrhythmias of the transplanted heart most commonly occur in the setting of acute cardiac allograft rejection. Thus, the treatment, directed toward rejection, is normally sufficient to control these arrhythmias. Procainamide and quinidine have been used successfully as antiarrhythmic agents in the transplant recipient.[3,6] The results of these earlier studies suggest that cardiac innervation is not an absolute requirement for a cardiac response to antiarrhythmic therapy with these agents.

β–adrenergic Blocking Agents

The denervated transplanted human heart is heavily dependent on circulating catecholamines during periods of stress.[10] The response to circulating catecholamines is also critical for exercise capacity and the heart rate response of transplant recipients.[5] Early in exercise, there is minimal change in heart rate with an increased stroke volume secondary to an increase in venous return. Later in exercise, there is an increase in heart rate due to circulating catecholamines. Thus the use of β blockers in transplant recipients may inhibit the major compensatory mechanisms of the denervated heart and may dramatically reduce the exercise tolerance of transplant patients. In addition, ß-blockers are negative inotropes and may potentially affect cardiac contractile function.

CARDIAC ALLOGRAFT REJECTION

Cardiac allograft rejection is a "natural" immunological complication of cardiac transplantation. Almost all transplant recipients develop at least a mild form of acute rejection. Cardiac allograft rejection can be divided into hyperacute, acute and chronic forms. Hyperacute rejection is a result of either the presence of preformed cytotoxic antibodies possessed by the recipient and directed towards donor lymphocytes or a mismatching of ABO blood groups. The diagnosis is usually obvious due to catastrophic problems manifested even in the operating room upon restoration of blood flow to the donor heart. This form of rejection is usually described as permanent and most frequently fatal. Intensive immunosuppressive therapy and inotropic support of the myocardium is essential in an attempt to salvage the heart. Aggressive treatment with very high doses of corticosteroids, high dose cyclophosphamide, and plasmapheresis may allow the patient to survive the initial event. However, the heart usually rapidly deteriorates despite all measures. The physical means to salvage this type of patient is the removal of the rejecting heart and the implementation of a total artificial heart while waiting for a second donor organ for retransplantation. The total artificial heart should facilitate the recovery of the patient and allow time to find a suitable donor with a negative lymphocyte cross match. Fortunately, this form of catastrophe is rare. With proper preoperative antibody screening and careful attention to blood typing, hyperacute rejection should fall in the less than 1% complication rate.

Acute rejection is the most common variety of rejection and in the majority of cases is caused by cell mediated processes. However, a humorally mediated form of acute vascular rejection has been described and is being recognized with increasing frequency. Chronic rejection usually refers to the development of allograft coronary atherosclerosis, which is felt to be the result of chronic immune mediated endothelial injury. This form of rejection is poorly understood and is still a hypothesis, still not proven and is not attenuated with immunosuppression augmentation. When advanced, this process leads to ischemic left ventricular dysfunction and ultimate graft failure.

Before the introduction of cyclosporine in 1980, a major cause of mortality in the immediate postoperative period was due to acute allograft rejection. Since the beginning of the "Cyclosporine Era," the mortality due to acute rejection has been substantially reduced. Although, in the majority of cases, acute rejection represents a single episode of rejection, several groups have noted vascular or cellular inflammation and/or damage occurring during cardiac allograft rejection carrying an adverse prognosis. This has been characterized as "vascular rejection." Herskowitz et al[13] have detailed the humoral rejection.

New onset arrhythmias, lethargy, gallops, pericardial friction rubs, low cardiac output, and decreased EKG voltage or other nonspecific and unexplained clinical findings should always be considered a possible manifestation of acute cardiac rejection in the initial days following transplantation. We and other transplant centers maintain a very low threshold for performance of endomyocardial biopsies as a means to diagnose acute rejection of the donor heart. The procedure is safe and is the most accurate means of detecting early rejection episodes, some occurring as early as three days post-transplantation. The majority of patients develop an average of one or two rejection episodes in the perioperative period.[1] Although new methods for noninvasive monitoring of rejection after heart transplantation are being rapidly developed, endomyocardial biopsy remains the "gold standard" for diagnosis of cardiac rejection. The noninvasive tests of potential value are Fast Fourier Transformed Serial Electrocardiography which determines the beat to beat variation by a power spectrum analysis and two-dimensional echocardiography. With 2-D echocardiography, mild to moderate rejection is associated with a significant decrease in left ventricular cross sectional area. Observations include changes in the diastolic maximum velocity, increased wall thickness, and in the case of acute severe rejection, reduction in left ventricular ejection fraction. Frequency analysis of surface ECG by FFT-ECG has a sensitivity of 95% although the exact specificity of this procedure remains unknown. Two-dimensional echocardiography is routinely used to aid in the diagnosis of acute allograft rejection with hemodynamic compromise. This diagnostic tool has the ability to serially determine the ventricular diastolic and systolic function and rule out the presence of significant pericardial effusion with tamponade as a cause for hemodynamic compromise.

Magnetic resonance imaging (MRI) with its excellent noninvasive morphological detail and tissue characterization is being applied to the problem of acute rejection. In animal models of acute cardiac allograft rejection the MRI signals especially those associated with cellular water content have been found to precede the histologic diagnosis of rejection. Similar results have been reported in small clinical studies and currently it would appear that a negative MRI study may obviate the need for endomyocardial biopsy. Precise specificity and cost effectiveness of MRI technology for the diagnosis of rejection still awaits careful, clinical investigation.[1]

HEART TRANSPLANT GRAFT ATHEROSCLEROSIS

Accelerated coronary atherosclerosis is the major cause of long-term graft failure and death in cardiac transplant patients despite improved immunosuppression and clinical management which have considerably enhanced long-term survival. (Fig.1) Graft atherosclerosis occurs in 40-78% of patients surviving five years.[1-4] The syndrome of accelerated coronary atherosclerosis leads to the familiar clinical sequelae of myocardial infarction, congestive heart failure, ventricular arrhythmias and sudden death often without symptoms of angina unless reinnervation of the transplanted heart has occurred. Thus the detection of progressive narrowing of the coronary arteries and ischemia necessitates frequent coronary angiograms. The overall prevalence of angiographically diagnosed coronary artery disease in transplanted hearts is significantly high: a rate of 10-20% at one year, 25-45% at three years, and 40-78% at 5 years.[16,17,1]

Cardiac transplant patients maintained on cyclosporine immunosuppression have a lower incidence of acute allograft rejection compared to patients being treated with azathioprine, but there is no decrease in the incidence of transplant coronary artery disease. In cardiac transplant patients on cyclosporine, coronary artery disease is not inhibited by the addition of antiplatelet drugs. Graft atherosclerosis is usually rapid in onset (months), usually silent and manifested by congestive heart failure or sudden death. Histopathologically there is diffuse involvement of the epicardial vessels, demonstrating concentric intimal proliferation consisting of smooth muscle cells and lymphocytes. The process is diffuse especially in the middle to distal vessels with some proximal lesions and severe distal vessel disease with very poor collaterals. The diffuse nature of this disease makes these patients poor candidates for angioplasty or bypass surgery, with re-transplantation being the present option. In contrast, native coronary artery disease, i.e. nonallograft, is slow in onset, occurs in the setting of known risk factors, and is manifested by angina. The coronary anatomy involves epicardial coronary arteries with focal and eccentric lesions which are often complex, histologically have lipids, macrophages, foam cells, scanty smooth muscle cells and are often associated with thrombi. This condition, unlike transplant atherosclerosis, is amenable to revascularization either by angioplasty, atherectomy or coronary bypass surgery.

Clinical Significance

Numerous studies have demonstrated that accelerated post-transplant coronary artery disease has a limited relationship to clinical and laboratory findings. The major correlates, although not definitely proven, have been reported to be higher donor age, elevated total cholesterol, triglycerides and rejection episodes. In one recent study increased body index (obesity) was the single most predictive risk factor for post-transplant coronary artery disease.[1] The degree of HLA mismatch and the type of immunosuppressive therapy do not consistently emerge as determinants of accelerated coronary artery disease. Standard interpretation of routine coronary angiography tends to underestimate the presence and severity of the distal vessel disease which often presents early after cardiac transplantation. In a 1989 study of 130 coronary angiograms in cardiac transplant patients performed at yearly intervals, Gao et al[16] demonstrated a 47% incidence of small vessel disease at one year in contrast to only 7% demonstrating discrete proximal lesions. These proximal lesions progressed over the year with an incidence of 75% at five to six years. These clinical observations suggest that post-transplant coronary artery disease at five years and later is a combination of small vessel disease due to immune mediated injury and typical atherosclerosis superimposed on this process due to the prevailing risk factors of hyperlipidemia and hypertension.

Accelerated coronary artery disease also occurs in pediatric heart transplant recipients, and is morphologically and clinically similar to that occurring in adults.[20] These lesions are frequently marked by subtle diffuse decreases in luminal area in adjacent segments. Relatively novel diagnostic strategies have been recently proposed which are based on endothelial derived relaxing factor (EDRF) mediated vasodilation to acetylcholine. Paradoxical vasoconstriction to acetylcholine suggests endothelial dysfunction or inactivation of endothelium dependent vasodilators. Impaired response to acetylcholine is a common early finding in heart transplant recipients and thus intracoronary acetylcholine may be useful in identifying early disease before overt angiographic abnormalities are observed. Intravascular ultrasound may also provide a unique approach to determining intimal thickening.

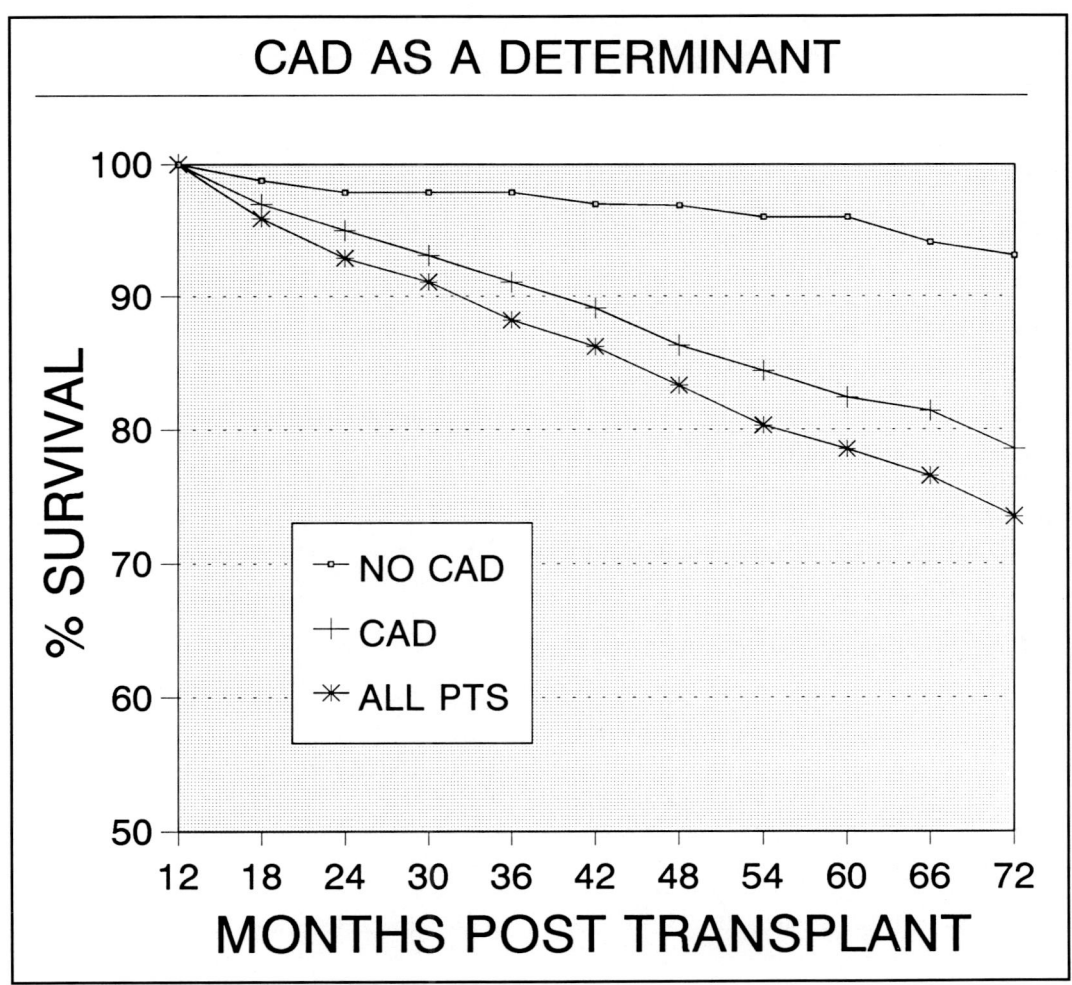

Fig.1. Long-term transplant survival.

Pathogenesis

The exact pathogenic mechanisms underlying the usual form of accelerated coronary artery disease after cardiac transplantation remains unclear. Ischemic injury to coronary endothelium before graft implantation, infection or reactivation of cytomegalovirus (CMV), hyperlipidemia or other host metabolic derangements due to immunosuppression, may all be contributing factors. However, the limited involvement of transplanted coronary arteries with sparing of host native vessels argues against a causal role for either systemic or metabolic effects of immunosuppressive agents or opportunistic infection in the development of accelerated coronary artery disease in the transplanted human heart. Thus an immunological process provoked by histocompatibility mismatch may explain the selective involvement of the coronary arteries of the transplanted human heart. Studies by Libby et al[24] suggest that when the recipient's immune cells, particularly T-lymphocytes, come in contact with endothelium of the grafted arteries, they are stimulated to release lymphokines, which modulate immunoreactions. In addition, the lymphokine, gamma interferon, can induce endothelial and smooth muscle cells to express immune molecules, known as a class II major histocompatibility proteins. Class II immunomolecules on the endothelial surface may induce a second wave of lymphokine producing immune cells, including macrophages which produce free radicals and other cytotoxic products. The resultant defect in the control of smooth muscle cell proliferation appears to cause the characteristic myointimal hyperplasia which is the key element in the obstructive lesions observed in the coronary arteries of transplant patients. It has been shown that endothelial injury induces putative mitogenic substances such as platelet derived growth factor, fibroblast growth factor and transforming growth factor which may contribute to smooth muscle cell migration and proliferation in the intima. On the other hand, lack of growth inhibitors such as heparin-like substances, normally produced by endothelial and smooth muscle cells, may also lead to abnormal regulation of smooth muscle cell proliferation.

Thus, the endothelial injury may be subtle and not detectable by ordinary histologic or angiographic examination. These endothelial injuries perhaps are altered physiologic states induced by chemical, physical or immunologic stimuli. Percutaneous transluminal coronary angioplasty is an everyday example of physically induced endothelial injury. The problem of restenosis, seen in 25% to 55% of patients by six months, is an all too well known occurrence. Histologic examination of these restenotic lesions demonstrates that intimal hyperplasia, secondary to smooth muscle cell proliferation, is the predominant component; not unlike the histopathology seen with accelerated transplant atherosclerosis. Here, as with transplant coronary disease, growth factors have been postulated to play an intricate role in the proliferative process.

In summary, post-transplant coronary atherosclerosis is an obstructive, proliferative lesion which is a major limiting factor in the long-term survival of cardiac transplant patients. This syndrome is typically insidious due to the diffuse nature of the lesions and lack of clinical symptoms. Although the exact mechanisms are unclear at present emerging data suggests that the primary insighting stimulus is an immune mediated coronary vascular injury.

SYSTEMIC HYPERTENSION

Systemic hypertension develops in a large majority of patients after heart transplantation and the immunosuppressive agent cyclosporine is believed to be an important contributor. However, the exact underlying mechanism of post-transplant hypertension is unknown. This form of hypertension occurs despite lower dosages of cyclosporine and in the absence of significant impairment of renal function. The factors which have been implicated in post-transplant hypertension include activation of the renin-angiotensin system, sympathetic neural activation, and effect of corticosteroids, particularly a mineralcorticoid effect resulting in a volume overload state and systemic arterial hypertension. The presence of normal cardiac filling pressures and cardiac output in the presence of hypertension does not support the concept of volume overload hypertension. Hypertension is universal and striking in patients receiving cyclosporine based triple immunosuppression or cyclosporine plus azathioprine. That fact along with the uncommon and mild findings in patients receiving conventional, i.e. azathioprine and prednisone, immunosuppression further suggest that corticosteroids have no significant role in the pathogenesis or cardiac transplant hypertension.

No definite neurohumoral abnormalities have been identified in cardiac transplant recipients that are responsible for the pathogenesis of post-transplant hypertension. Studies by Olivari et al[27] have concluded that levels of plasma norepinephrine return to normal within six months after cardiac transplantation. Thompson et al[28] measured upright renin and 24-hour urinary catecholamines in transplant recipients and concluded that there were no abnormalities in a group of cyclosporine treated patients. Similarly, all clinical studies have concluded that the renin-aldosterone and angiotensin axis are within normal limits under base line conditions. Myers et al[29] studied a group of cyclosporine and non-cyclosporine treated cardiac transplant recipients one year after transplantation. In cyclosporine treated patients, active renin was strikingly lower while inactive renin was high. These results led this group to conclude that long-term cyclosporine therapy may cause partial blocking of the intrarenal conversion of inactive renin to active renin. Atrial natriuretic peptide levels have been reported to be high in cardiac transplant recipients two years following cardiac transplantation but no correlation has been observed between the arterial pressure and levels of atrial natriuretic peptide.

The pathophysiologic mechanisms of cyclosporine treated post-transplant hypertension are unclear. In ambulatory heart transplant recipients, the hypertensive effect of cyclosporine has been demonstrated most vividly. The incidence of hypertension has increased from less than 20% in the pre-cyclosporine era to now, better than 90%. This hypertension typically is moderate to severe and often requires multiple antihypertensive agents for treatment. Hypertension has become one of the most important problems in the medical management of heart transplant recipients. In anesthetized animal preparations, acute administration of cyclosporine stimulates sympathetic outflow. In heart transplant recipients, this effect of cyclosporine might be accentuated because cardiac transplantation interrupts the afferent (as well as efferent) neural connections from the transplanted ventricles to the central nervous system and thus removes ventricular baroreceptor restraint on sympathetic outflow. Scherrer et al,[31] demonstrated that cyclosporine is a potent stimulus to sympathetic nerve activity in humans. Their studies demonstrated that the sympathetic discharge of hypertensive heart transplant recipients taking cyclosporine, azathioprine and prednisone was three times higher than in normal controls. In contrast, the level of sympathetic discharge was normal in normotensive heart transplant recipients who were taking prednisone and azathioprine without cyclosporine. Also of note, there was no difference in sympathetic activity (discharge) in patients with essential hypertension and patients not on cyclosporine. Patients with myasthenia gravis on cyclosporine also have significant increases in arterial pressure and in sympathetic discharge which might indicate that although sympathetic activation during cyclosporine administration is not dependent on denervation such denervation may augment the stimulation of sympathetic outflow evoked by cyclosporine. In this study, the myasthenic patients taking cyclosporine had normal norepinephrine levels but were 50% higher than transplant patients not on cyclosporine. These abnormal levels are associated with significant sympathetic discharge. Thus normal urinary and serum norepinephrine levels cannot exclude increased sympathetic discharge as the etiology of hypertension in patients on cyclosporine. Comparable doses of cyclosporine cause larger increases in both sympathetic activity and blood pressure in heart transplant recipients than in the patients with myasthenia gravis and normally innervated hearts. While many different mechanisms are likely to be involved in the pathogenesis of cyclosporine induced hypertension, the neurophysiologic data of Scherrer provides one potential explanation for the clinical observation that the hypertensive effect of cyclosporine tends to be greater in heart transplant patients than in other groups of patients.

It has been suggested that impairment of renal function may be a factor in hypertension after transplantation. Multiple adverse effects of cyclosporine on renal function have been described. They include a reversible dose-dependent increase in serum creatine and disproportionate increase in blood urea nitrogen, hypokalemia, metabolic acidosis, hyperchloremia, type 4 renal tubular acidosis and chronic interstitial nephritis with irreversible renal toxicity.[26,1,2] The mechanisms involved in cyclosporine renal toxicity are unclear but experimental evidence favors tubular toxicity, vasomotor effects of cyclosporine on the renal blood vessels and a specific cyclosporine associated vascular lesion.

Cardiac transplant hypertension is often severe and refractory to multiple antihypertensive drug regimens. The drugs that have been utilized successfully include angiotensin converting enzyme inhibitors, calcium channel blockers, β blockers and α blocking agents. To date, there are no randomized clinical trials examining the effectiveness of various pharmacologic strategies in the treatment of post-transplant hypertension. Our experience and the experience of other transplant centers indicate that post-transplant hypertension can be refractory and optimal control is often difficult to achieve despite the use of multiple potent antihypertensive drugs. Our experience and the experience of others, however, suggest nifedipine XL in combination with diuretics is often effective in achieving reasonable control of the hypertension, at least during the early post-transplant period. Severe hypertension refractory to long-acting nifedipine and diuretics may respond to the addition of angiotensin converting enzyme inhibitors to this regimen.

The evidence thus far presented suggests that post-transplant hypertension is in part cyclosporine-induced and that the cardiac denervation that occurs with cardiac transplantation may augment the magnitude of this hypertension. The universal occurrence of hypertension and its refractory nature often leads to left ventricular hypertrophy with evidence of diastolic ventricular dysfunction. Long-standing hypertension and left ventricular hypertrophy may ultimately lead to a hypertensive cardiomyopathy similar to that observed in the nontransplanted hypertensive population. In order to avoid the long-term morbidity and mortality associated with cyclosporine induced hypertension, early and aggressive treatment of hypertension will be necessary.

FUTURE TRENDS AND CHALLENGES

The decade of the 80s brought us the era of cyclosporine immunosuppression. Together with increasing knowledge, careful patient selection, and overall refinement of technical skills, this resulted in a very achievable goal of over a 90% one-year survival rate in cardiac transplantation. Indeed, this was a significant advance but it did produce a double-edged sword in our patients. It would appear that our patients traded very aggressive rejection that was observed in the patients maintained on a conventional prednisone-azathioprine protocol, and gave us in return the long-term problems of hypertension and chronic renal insufficiency. Even this present 10% one-year mortality rate should be amenable to further reduction in the future. The goal will be the discovery and creation of better myocardial preservation and better cardioplegia enabling longer ischemic times in conjunction with improved postoperative performance of the transplanted heart. This, indeed, is an active area of investigation and hopefully will result in an increased better functioning donor organ supply.

Acute rejection and the infectious complications long the nemesis in the battleground of the first year post-cardiac transplantation indeed appear to be controllable disease entities. With the emergence of newer and hopefully better immunosuppression on the horizon acute rejection appears to be under control. The elusive search for the noninvasive diagnosis of acute rejection continues, but the gold standard of endomyocardial biopsy continues to remain the transplanter's best friend. The potential of such technology as Fast Fourier Transformed Serial Electrocardiography, two-dimensional echocardiography, and magnetic resonance imaging exists. This technology may make the diagnosis of acute rejection possible on the examining table in the transplant clinic. This, indeed, will be a step forward in both the rapidity of diagnosis and a further reduction in the cost of diagnosis of acute rejection. Current treatment protocols with pulsed methylprednisolone are decreasing the dose utilized so successfully in the past. It is heartening to see smaller doses of methylprednisolone accomplishing the desired result. Perhaps in the future multiple additions of immunosuppressive agents in terms of combinations of FK506, Rapamycin and cyclosporine, whether it be A or G, may result in the further reduction in steroid requirements. The pioneering work of the Utah group and the Medical College of Virginia group in the mid-1980s declaring long-term prednisone to be an unacceptable alternative in cardiac transplantation will be continued. With the development of improved immunosuppression, it would appear that prednisone will become a historical drug and the infectious complications along with "metabolic complications" of prednisone therapy will be eliminated. Indeed, this should be encouraged and promoted.

The double-edged sword of hypertension and chronic renal insufficiency created by cyclosporine hopefully will be significantly reduced or eliminated with the development of improved immunosuppression. The very intriguing tool of diltiazem used with cyclosporine, decreasing the total dosage of cyclosporine, and still offering optimal immunosuppression can serve as a harbinger of things to come. Our second generation immunosuppressive agents hopefully will result in a further decrease in hypertension and chronic renal insufficiency.

The remaining problem of accelerated coronary artery disease is, indeed, the challenge of the 1990s. In the area of diagnosis, significant progress has been made. Our current gold standard remains the coronary angiogram which admittedly can lead to false negative results and is at best difficult to interpret. Already the concept of coronary artery responsiveness is gaining much better acceptance and in the future we may indeed be making the diagnosis not by sitting in front of the viewbox but by examining the data and the results of coronary flow reserve studies. Further, it will only be a short time until coronary artery ultrasound is applied to the cardiac transplant recipient. Indeed, this will be able to directly diagnose luminal narrowing without the pitfalls of angiography.

The treatment of accelerated coronary artery disease is the single most challenging problem for the future. It would appear with cardiac transplantation that we are basically watching the heart age in front of us. What takes years to decades to develop as coronary atherosclerosis in the native heart appears to be accelerated into terms of weeks to months in the transplanted heart. Our current understanding is pitifully small. We can make inroads in the known risk factors and apply our knowledge of risk factor modification presently to our patients and thereby modify Type I vascular injury to a degree. There should be no cardiac transplant recipient permitted to smoke cigarettes, and the hypertension of cardiac transplantation should be aggressively treated. Lipid abnormalities in terms of hypercholesterolemia should be aggressively treated. The recent safe formulation of the use of Lovastatin in combination with cyclosporine appears to be promising. Long-term trials are needed to see that if the low dose Lovastatin with the subsequent 20-30% decrease in total cholesterol values can, indeed, delay the onset of accelerated coronary atherosclerosis. The new second generation, coenzyme A reductase inhibitors should be carefully screened and evaluated in our patient population to see if they offer: 1) a decrease in interaction with cyclosporine, and 2) optimal control of the patient's lipid status, and 3) inhibition of the accelerated coronary atherosclerosis process. Obviously, the problem of obesity should be aggressively managed and diabetes controlled extremely carefully. Percutaneous transluminal coronary angioplasty indeed will remain a pallative therapy for patients who develop fixed proximal obstructive disease as seen in the later years post-cardiac transplantation. The application of either laser angioplasty or coronary atherectomy has already been applied to car-

Table 1.

Complications	1992	1993 and Beyond
Rejection (acute)		
•Diagnosis	Endomyocardial biopsy	Fast Fourier transformed serial electrocardiography Two-dimentional echocardiography
•Treatment	Pulsed-methyl prednisolone	FK-406 Rapamycin
•Hypertension	Diltiazem Nifedipine ACE Inhibitors	Second generation ACE inhibitors Renin antagonist Calcium channel blockers
Chronic (Accelerated CAD)		
Treatment	•Risk factor modification •cigarettes •hypertension •diabetes •lipids •obesity •PTCA	Lovastatin
Diagnosis	Angiography	Coronary artery responsiveness Coronary artery ultrasound

diac transplant patients with accelerated coronary atherosclerosis. The success of these techniques awaits verification. Still, aggressive modification of risk factors and the palliation of mechanical coronary artery procedures will not keep the coronary tree from aging in front of us. Further diligent investigation is absolutely necessary to understand this basic process so that we can map out the molecular mechanisms involved and, hopefully, design pharmacology capable of inhibiting this process and significantly retarding and/or eliminating the development of what still appears to be the rate-limiting step in cardiac transplantation, that is, accelerated coronary atherosclerosis. This, indeed, is the challenge for the 1990s. (Table 1)

ACKNOWLEDGEMENT

This work was performed during the tenure of the Merck/American College of Cardiology Fellowship to Dr. David E. Tolman. Supported in part by Grant-in-Aid RR00065 to the Clinical Research Center of the Medical College of Virginia.

The authors would like to thank Dr. Michael Kaye, Editor, *Journal of Heart and Lung Transplantation*, for his help in providing the data from the International Registry for Figure 1.

References

1. Corcos T, Tamburino C, Leger P et al. Early and late hemodynamic evaluation after cardiac transplantation. J Am Coll of Cardiol 1988; 11:264-9.
2. Borow KM, Newman A, Arensman FW, Yaconie MH. Left ventricular contractility and contractile reserve in humans after cardiac transplantation. Circ 1985; 71:866-72.
3. Schroeder JS, Gerke DK, Graham AF, Rider AK, Harrison DC. Arrhythmias after heart transplantation. Am J Cardiol 1974; 33:604-610.
4. Romhilt DW, Doyle M, Sagar KB et al. Prevalence and significance of arrhythmias in long-term survival of cardiac transplantation. Circ 1982; 66 (Suppl I):219-226.
5. Bexton RS, Nathan AW, Hellerstrand KJ et al. Electrophysiologic abnormalities in the transplanted human heart. Br Heart J 1983; 50:555-561.
6. Berke DK, Graham AF, Schroeder JS, Harrison DC. Arrhythmias in the devervated transplanted human heart. Circ 1978; 47 Cardiovasc Surg (Suppl III):112-118.
7. Sands KF, Appel ML, Lily LS, Schoen FJ, Mudge GH, Cohen RJ. Powerspectrum analysis of heart rate variability in cardiac transplant recipients. Circ 1989; 79:76-82.
8. Stark RP, McGinn AL, Wilson RF. Chest pain in cardiac-transplant recipients. Evidence of sensory reinnervation after cardiac transplantation. New Eng J Med 1991; 324:1791-4.
9. Schroeder JS, Gao S-Z, Alderman EL, Hunt SA, Stinson E. Diltiazem inhibits development of early accelerated transplant coronary disease: An interim report. Abstract: American Heart Association Scientific Sessions; 1990.
10. Mohanty PK, Sowers JR, Thames MD, Beck FWJ, Kawaguchi A, Lower RR. Myocardial norepinephrine, epinephrine and dopamine concentrations after cardiac auto-transplantation in dogs. J Am Coll Cardiol 1986; 7:419-24.
11. Donald DE, Shepherd JT. Supersensitivity to l-norepinephrine the denervated sinoatrial node. Am J Physiol 1965; 208:255-9.
12. Ebert PA. The effects of norepinephrine infusion on the denervated heart. J of Cardiovasc Surg 1968; 9:414-19.
13. Herskowitz A, Soule LM, Ueda K et al. Arteriolar vaculitis on endomyocardial biopsy: A histologic predictor of poor outcome in cyclosporine-treated heart transplant recipients. J Heart Transplant 1987; 6:127-36.
14. Bollman RM, Elick B, Olivari M-T et al. Improved immunosuppression for heart transplantation. J Heart Transplant 1985; 4:315-19.
15. Wisenburg G, Pflugfekler PW, Kostud et al. Diagnostic applicability of magnetic resonance imaging in assessing human cardiac allograft rejection. Am J Cardiol 1987:60:130-6.
16. Gao S-Z, Schroeder JS, Alderman EL, Silverman JF, Hunt SA. Accelerated coronary vascular disease in the heart transplant patient. Coronary arteriographic findings. J Am Coll Cardiol 1988:12:334-340.
17. Uretsky BF, Murah S, Reddy RS et al. Development of coronary artery disease in cardiac transplant patients receiving immunosuppressive therapy with cyclosporine and prednisone. Circ 1987; 76:827-834.
18. Hess ML, Hastillo A, Thompson JA et al. Lipid mediators in organ transplantation-Does cyclosporine accelerate coronary atherosclerosis? Transplant Proc 1987; 19 (Suppl 5):71-3.
19. Taylor DO, Ibrahim HM, Tolman DE, Hess ML. Accelerated coronary atherosclerosis in cardiac transplantation. Trans Rev 1991; 5:165-174.
20. Pahl E, Frucker FJ, Armitage J et al. Coronary atherosclerosis in pediatric heart transplant survivors: Limitaiton of long-term survival. J Pediatr 1990; 116:177-193.
21. Winters GL, Kendall TJ, Radio SJ et al. Post transplant obesity and hyperlipidemia: Major prediction of severity of coronary arteriopathy in failed human heart allografts. J Heart Transplant 1990; 9:364-371.
22. Gao S-Z, Schroeder JS, Alderman El et al. Prevalence of accelerated coronary artery disease in heart transplant survivors. Comparison of cyclosporine and azathioprine regimens. Circ 1989; 80(suppl3):III 100-105.
23. Fish RD, Nabel EG, Selwyn AP et al. Response of coronary arteries of cardiac transplant patients to acetycholine. J Clin Invest 1988; 81:21-31.
24. Libby P, Salomon RN, Payne DD, Schoen FJ, Pober JS. functions of vascular wall cells related to development of transplantation associated coronary atherosclerosis. Transplant Proc 1989; 4:3677-84.
25. Cercek B, Sharifi B, Barath P, Bailey L, Forrester JS. Growth factors in pathogenesis of coronary arterial restenosis. Am J Cardio 1991; 68:24C-33C.
26. Myers BD, Ross J, Newton L, Luetscher J, Perlroth M. Cyclosporine associated chronic nephropathy. New Eng J Med 1984; 311:699-705.
27. Olivari M-T, Levine TB, Ring WS, Simon A, Cohn JN. Normalization of sympathetic nervous system function after orthotopic cardiac transplant in man. Circ 1987; 76:62-4.
28. Thompson ME, Shapiro AP, Johnsen AM et al. New onset of hypertension following cardiac transplantation: A preliminary report and analysis. Transplant Proc 1983; 15(suppl1):2573.
29. Myers BD, Ross J, Newton L, Luetscher J, Perlroth M. Cyclosporine associated chronic nephropathy. New Eng J Med 1984; 311:699-705.
30. Seehan HM, Graham S, Hodgson JM, Ellenbogen KA, Mohanty PK. Influence of hypertension and coronary artery disease on left ventricular function after heart transplantation. Clin Res 1990; 38:336A.
31. Scherrer U, Vissing SF, Morgan BJ, Ring S, Hanson P, Mohanty PK, Victor R. Cyclosporine induced sympathetic activation and hypertension after heart transplantation. N Eng J Med 1990; 323:693-699.
32. Kahan BD. Cyclosporine nephrotoxicity pathogenesis, prophylaxis therapy and prognosis. Am J of Kidney Dis 1986; 8:3230-31.
33. Murray BM, Paller MS, Ferris TF. Effect of cyclosporine on renal hemodynamics in conscious rats. Kidney Internl 1985; 28:767-74.

CHAPTER 5

MEDICAL COMPLICATIONS OF LUNG TRANSPLANTATION

R. Scott Stuart

William A. Baumgartner

INTRODUCTION

The occurrence of significant complications subsequent to any operative procedure is at best demoralizing to the patient and the surgeon and at worse, a life threatening event. Certainly transplantation stands as an area of great risk for complications and nowhere is the tight rope higher for potential disastrous complications than in lung transplantation. Of all currently common transplants, it is the only organ which is in constant contact with the "outside world" and thus most at risk for potential problems such as aspiration and infection, both in the donor or the recipient. Furthermore, when graft failure occurs there is no current means for adequately temporizing graft function until treatment and healing occurs or retransplantation is undertaken. This fact, combined with the need for immediate and continued adequate lung function for the patient, creates a situation where any significant complication can quickly become magnified and life threatening.

As all physicians know, an exhaustive list of complications for any operative procedure can become endless if all possibilities are taken to their illogical extremes. The same is true for lung transplantation. Basically, however, there are six major risks which are currently encountered in this field. In order of usual appearance after transplantation, they are: (1) early graft failure secondary to inadequate preservation, (2) postoperative hemorrhage, (3) medication-induced renal impairment and or failure, (4) difficulties with the airway anastomoses (either early leak or late stenosis), (5) infection and (6) rejection: acute and chronic, the latter manifested as bronchiolitis obliterans.

This chapter will discuss each of the above risks with an eye toward future trends and will do so by first exploring ways to avoid the occurrence of the problem. The best way to treat any complication is to avoid it in the first place.

Further discussion will then entertain ways to treat the difficulty once it has risen.

PRESERVATION (OR THE LACK THEREOF!)

It is not too strong a statement to say that a properly selected and preserved lung would dramatically decrease many post-transplant complications which are currently encountered. Any physician who has had even a brief encounter with lung transplantation knows the all too familiar domino effect of a poorly preserved (or selected) lung which fails to provide good function at the time of re-anastomosis in the recipient. The scenario of reperfusion, pulmonary edema, difficulty with ventilation, poor oxygenation, and increasing airway pressures can rapidly lead to treatment therapies which can compromise multiple organ systems, most notably cardiac and renal. One could avoid such difficulties by (a) being able to improve donor selection and (b) improving lung preservation itself.

Donor Selection

Currently physicians are relatively limited in their ability to adequately assess and select a donor lung. Analyses of blood gases, sputum gram stains, serial chest x-rays, bronchoscopy, and visual inspection are all currently employed in evaluating a donor lung. However, such evaluations are quite crude and are frequently too insensitive to pick up early but potentially lethal problems within the donor lung which will express themselves only after implantation.

It is potentially possible to evaluate a donor lung for aspiration by use of technology which is currently available. This specifically relates to pH probes which may be passed through the biopsy channel of any standard bronchoscope. Such information would be useful should the pH of the distal airways prove to be acidotic even though visual inspection of those airways appears to be normal. Secondly, the lung is certainly more than a large inert bag for gas exchange and the use of metabolic markers may prove to be quite valuable in assessing lung function. Several animal studies over recent years have tried to exploit the lung's unique ability to

metabolize chemicals such as serotonin or angiotensin on a first pass basis. Such analyses are currently quite cumbersome but further advances may yield relatively simple laboratory techniques for the evaluation of serum levels of metabolites from serotonin or angiotensin. It is conceivable that small amounts of these drugs could be injected on the venous side, perhaps through a central line, with samples being withdrawn from the arterial side.

Newer and more efficient means for imaging would be invaluable. For example, even with the current models of magnetic resonance imaging devices, pulmonary vascular flow may be crudely but reasonably evaluated. As more efficient and accurate models of MRI systems become available, it is conceivable that any given donor could be easily evaluated for subtle changes in flow which could reflect potential areas of compromise due to aspiration, infection or contusion. Obviously, such evaluation would be limited to major centers.

Donor pulmonary emboli have certainly proven to be a very real, though, not easily documented entity which subsequently prevents adequate preservation by any method which employs intravascular flushing or perfusion. Improved imaging could potentially be the key to ferreting out this disastrous complication.

Improved Preservation

The current major methods of preservation employ either pulmonary artery flush or core-cooling. Preservation solutions are currently relatively crude and simply rely on intra- or extracellular compositions combined with hypothermia. This is adequate for reliable preservation between four - seven hours, but the ultimate goals for preservation are actually two in number: (1) achieving excellent preservation of all vascular endothelium and bronchial epithelium and (2) that such preservation may be adequate for extended hours or potentially even days. This situation would allow not only for daylight implantations but more importantly provide the ability to accurately match donor and recipient, and thereby minimize or avoid another major complication: rejection. Numerous studies are in progress investigating various additives which either limit or completely prevent the difficulties which occur in the "final common pathways to injury". Such theories revolve around the production and damage caused by oxygen free radicals and lipid peroxidation. There is a large body of data supporting the concept and use of free radical scavengers. These scavengers include superoxide dismutase, catalase, deferoxamine and DMSO. In addition techniques to minimize the free radical cascade could provide benefit. Specifically, this refers to the augmentation of the free radical effect by leukocytes, and certainly very promising research is currently underway which may lead to the clinical application of leukocyte filters which could be employed in the procurement of a donor lung and its subsequent implantation into the recipient.

In the realm of lipid peroxidation and its deleterious side effects on membrane integrity, new drugs which fall into the general categories of cerebrosides and lazaroids are providing other interventional agents to use against one of the arms of what is certainly three or four pillars of the "final common pathway". Such cellular injury patterns are multifactorial but a potential preservation "cocktail" might combine elements of free radical scavengers, antilipid peroxidants and other agents to directly decrease the tendency towards capillary leak, e.g. nitric oxide analogues which directly affect endothelium cell relaxing factor. The best method for delivering such a solution remains in question. Pulmonary artery flush has shown itself to be a simple tool for preservation. Nonetheless it does share the same problem with preservation flushes for other organs, in that a small but real obligate time of warm ischemia does exist. The technique of core-cooling has as its advantage the ability to deliver high volumes of fluid through a simplified cardiopulmonary bypass system which allows for: hemodynamic stability, gradual cooling, the easy addition of additives to a preservation solution, the ability to employ a leukocyte filter, and with the new heparinless cardiopulmonary systems which are currently coming on the market, problems of augmented inflammation and

capillary leak should be dramatically decreased.

At Implantation

Once the lung procurement team returns to the recipient hospital and the implantation begins, there are two areas for improvement which should be stressed. The first is technical and relates to the development of an effective, yet technically facile method for reimplantation of the bronchial arteries. With the current techniques, the new grafts do perform relatively well, but there is no doubt that the reimplantation of a bronchial artery with subsequent arterialized blood flow to all regions of the new graft would increase the chances for improved function. The second improvement relates to cellular function itself. With the ischemia time and subsequent revascularization with reduced oxygenated blood, the type II alveolar cells suffer a decrease in their function and efficiency. Very encouraging evidence exists for the use of externally applied surfactant (delivered via the airway) as evidenced in the current use of this drug in Neonatal Intensive Care Units. Certainly surfactant, which resides within the alveoli at the time of transplantation, must be compromised by ischemia and atelectasis. Further, the type II alveolar cells are not able to adequately and quickly produce new surfactant. The ability to supply external surfactant which would be capable of reaching lower airways and alveoli could be invaluable to overcome the surface tension which leads to alveolar collapse. Externally supplied surfactant which is given to neonates with immature lungs has yielded dramatic results. It would be hoped that similar success would be achieved in a more developed adult organ.

TREATING PRESERVATION FAILURES

The next question arises as to what to do with a poorly preserved lung if postimplantation pulmonary edema develops despite the best efforts of both donor and recipient teams. Currently, aggressive use of diuretics and increasing ventilatory support are employed. The usual outcome, however, is worsening airway pressures with subsequent airway damage which only intensifies a vicious cycle towards graft failure. Furthermore, aggressive use of diuretics combined with nephrotoxic immunosuppressive medications, such as cyclosporine or FK506, produce renal impairment and occasionally ATN.

Basically the lung needs time to heal after suffering an ischemic/reperfusion injury and profound capillary leak. Such remodeling and healing can occur but the time needed is directly proportional to the degree of preservation injury. Relatively minor degrees of preservation injury may require only 24-48 hours for reversal of capillary leak. However, such rapid repair is not always possible when aggressive ventilatory management, higher FiO_2s, and increasing airway pressures are needed to sustain life. Therefore what is needed is essentially an artificial lung to support the patient. Currently, the only feasible option is the existence of ECMO. Obviously, this has proven to be difficult in that total heparinization has been traditionally required due to the oxygenator within the circuit. However, with new heparinless systems becoming available, long periods of circulatory and gas exchange support are potentially feasible with minimal or no heparin. Support times of several days to weeks look to be possible within the next one to two years, let alone what may be achieved by the year 2000. Beyond the decrease in need for heparinization and subsequent decrease in bleeding, these systems are expected to dramatically decrease or eliminate the profound problems encountered with prolonged perfusion such as whole body inflammatory response and capillary leak within all major organ systems, including the lung.

Additionally, prototypes of intravascular oxygenating systems currently exist. These devices, which resemble the internal aspect of the membrane oxygenator but without its casing, are placed intravascularly within the venous system. Though they are most efficient in reducing carbon dioxide content, newer and more advanced models will be capable of supporting oxygenation. Such systems essentially allow the lung to be put to rest. Ventilators, per se, are used only at minimal settings in both rate and airway pressures. The lung indeed will remodel over time, even

following a severe preservation injury. A recent experience (RSS) involved a single lung transplant recipient who sustained a severe preservation injury due to unknown pulmonary emboli. This precluded adequate preservation at the time of procurement and resulted in severe injury. The patient underwent traditional ventilation which prolonged and worsened the airway component of the injury, but the lung progressively recovered over the ensuing six months to approximately 80% of its potential.

BLEEDING

Bleeding is a potential complication for any operative procedure, but in lung transplantation postoperative hemorrhage presents a serious threat to perioperative survival. Hemorrhage results in unstable hemodynamics as well as multiple blood product infusions leading to additional lung damage superimposed on the ischemic injury. Prevention of hemorrhage is a combination of recipient selection and meticulous hemostasis. The current use of argon beam lasers has been quite advantageous in lung transplant recipients requiring cardiopulmonary bypass for the completion of the procedure. Future advances in lasers and "hot knives" will allow for finer dissection without extensive tissue destruction. Furthermore, newer surgical techniques such as the use of a clam shell incision for bilateral lung transplantation will continue to improve results. Such incisions provide better access to difficult areas such as the apices of the lung and thus allow for better control of potential adhesions. As mentioned previously, the newer heparinless bypass circuits should dramatically improve the ability to minimize blood lost during and after bypass runs. The use of these new circuits with markedly reduced heparin levels and the resultant decrease in inflammatory response often initiated by current bypass circuits will be a major advance. Finally, new drugs such as aprotinin, which is currently used in Europe and being investigated in this country, show great promise for minimalization of postoperative hemorrhage, subsequent use of blood products and the attendant deleterious effects on graft function.

RENAL INSUFFICIENCY AND FAILURE

Recipients who are properly chosen for any transplantation procedure other than renal transplantation ideally should not have pre-existing renal insufficiency or renal failure. Renal complications encountered postoperatively are due to the recipient status, perioperative hemodynamic instability, and drug reactions which can induce renal failure, such as antibiotics and the immunosuppression drugs cyclosporine and FK506. Avoidance of this latter cause will occur with the emergence of future immunosuppressive drugs which do not have renal toxicity.

Renal insufficiency or failure following transplantation requires standard treatment modalities. Traditional dialysis can be employed if the patient is hemodynamically stable. If however, there are difficulties with fluid balance and hemodynamic instability the options of continuous arterial-venous hemodialysis or continuous ultrafiltration are the most useful techniques. In those patients who are hemodynamically unstable and additionally have problems with arterial access for dialysis, the option of veno-veno dialysis with an in-line bio-head pump is an excellent option. This will become increasingly useful with the newer forms of heparinless tubing and pump heads which are emerging now in the North American market.

AIRWAY COMPLICATIONS

Difficulties with airway anastomoses may be encountered on an acute or chronic basis. Acutely, these difficulties will present as either a peribronchial abscess secondary to an anastomotic leak or as an outright bronchopleural fistula. The size of such leaks can be exceedingly small or as problematic as a full dehiscence. The etiology of this complication is generally poor healing. This occurs secondary to a variety of causes including poor vascularity and rejection. Since the bronchial circulation is not reestablished, bronchial and tracheal anastomoses are at an increased ischemic risk. Rejection itself can cause vascular compromise by thrombosis of the smaller and more fragile terminal vessels at the bronchial connection. Therefore, a combination of improvements are necessary to decrease the number and severity of airway anastomotic problems. A variety of wraps including pericardial fat, intercostal muscle, internal mammary pedicle, and omentum have been employed with varying degrees of success. The operative technique itself would be advanced by the use of a laser assisted anastomosis which could meld the donor and recipient tissue planes into one continuous sheet and minimize the chance for subsequent leak. Additionally, improvements in immunosuppressive drugs which would reduce acute and chronic rejection would vastly improve the successful reestablishment of the microcirculation. Significant investigation into the application of angiogenic factors either as topical agents or as intravascular drugs is being actively pursued.

Chronic airway changes usually present as varying degrees of airway stenosis. They typically are treated by either reoperation or the use of intraluminal stents, usually being made of silastic material. The development of new conduits as either interpositions for the anastomosis itself or as stents would certainly facilitate the treatment of this potentially very difficult complication. Specifically, these conduits would be envisioned to be of living material and perhaps could even be constructed of bronchial cartilage which has been laboratory produced.

Technical advancements will make the anastomosis of the bronchial arteries a more realistic goal. Current techniques for harvesting and re-implantation for the bronchials are certainly possible, but are proving to be extraordinarily cumbersome and time consuming. Certainly with improvement in the microvascular technique, the direct anastomosis of the bronchials will become a reality and should lead to improved vascularity at the site of the anastomosis resulting in a decrease in acute dehiscence and chronic stenoses.

INFECTION

Preventing infection remains the ultimate goal in transplant recipients. This begins with adequate and improved means of evaluating the donor. Mention has already been made of the potential to evaluate the distal airways of donors with pH probes. Acidotic results would lead one to make a diagnosis of subtle aspiration and thus initiate prompt treatment or avoid using the lung. Certainly improved preservation of the lung as was discussed in an earlier aspect of the chapter, will provide more normal function and avoid areas of compromise following reperfusion. Thus, improved blood flow and oxygenation will reduce pulmonary infectious compromise and also provide for increased vascular access for prophylactic antibiotics. Certainly more specific immunosuppression directed to subsets of T-cell populations would be advantageous by allowing full neutrophil activity in fighting infection. The route of administration could also potentially increase the efficacy and potency of available antibiotics. The improved ability to aerosolize antibiotics would allow antibiotics to penetrate into the alveolar regions themselves. In terms of treatment, newer generations of antibiotics will undoubtedly continue to emerge. CMV pneumonitis has traditionally been associated with significant morbidity and mortality. The advent and clinical use of acyclovir and ganciclovir has allowed successful treatment of this disease. As CMV testing becomes more widely available, the ability to know the CMV status preoperatively will enhance the ability of transplant teams to seromatch CMV donors and recipients. Finally, in regards to the AIDS virus, obviously, only a full vaccine will give adequate protection against this potentially devastating disease.

REJECTION

The approach to limiting rejection in the postoperative period is really three-pronged. The first is to improve methods to decrease rejection in general, the second is to improve the methods for the diagnosis of acute and chronic rejection, and finally, the development of a more effective treatment regimen of rejection.

Prevention
The most effective way to avoid rejection is to closely match recipient and donor. Such detailed matching, even with currently available techniques, is a time-consuming affair. Such matching would require successful preservation of organs for 24-48 hours, similar to kidneys. However, even if available, this type of matching would require national sharing of organs, which would represent a major organizational change from the transplant activities currently employed. A potential method to increase donor organs is through xenotransplantation. Theoretically, such methods as genetic engineering could be employed to provide a similar HLA framework in an animal, such as a pig.

Improved immunosuppressive drugs given before and during the transplant procedure would provide for suppression of the immune system in a more efficient and selective fashion such that overall rejection would be decreased without the deleterious side effects which exist with currently available drugs. The ultimate goal of immunosuppression would be to induce tolerance within the recipient. Whether this is achieved by an immunosuppressive drug, or by vehicles such as antibody masking of donor antigens is unclear at this time. Tolerance could also potentially be induced by total lymphoid irradiation (TLI). Preliminary studies have shown the efficacy of TLI in the treatment of patients with severe ongoing rejection. Rejection episodes have been arrested, and future rejection episodes appear to be minimal or even absent.

Diagnosis
Transbronchial and open lung biopsy still remain the gold standard for diagnosing acute and chronic rejection in lung transplantation. Since these techniques are associated with morbidity and patient discomfort, a noninvasive method to detect rejection would be quite beneficial. This might entail a blood marker (perhaps as a side effect of T-cell or B-cell activity) or studies such as primed lymphocyte testing as espoused by the University of Pittsburgh group. Additionally, imaging itself might provide more information. It is possible that advanced editions of magnetic resonance imaging could provide sufficient data to diagnose rejection at an earlier stage. Tagged antibodies may be developed which would be specific for T-cell subsets which

predominate in rejection. Thus, periodic scans performed routinely or prompted by a clinical change might provide the opportunity to detect early rejection.

Treatment

The treatment of rejection needs to be more effective with fewer side effects. Furthermore, the effectiveness of the drug should ideally provide for a prolonged period of remission between potential rejection episodes. The ideal agent would be one that will specifically target those T-cell subsets which are responsible for rejection yet not affect the remaining T-cells, B-cells, neutrophils, and macrophages which are important to the infectious limb of the immune mechanism. Additionally, total lymphoid irradiation is being used more frequently. It is entirely conceivable that smaller doses applied at earlier stages in the postoperative course may prove to be quite useful in limiting or eliminating episodes of acute, recurrent, or chronic rejection.

New delivery systems for immunosuppressive drugs would certainly improve the opportunity to effectively treat rejection. Alternative methods of delivery such as finely aerosolized immunosuppressive drugs might allow for better delivery, absorption, and distribution of the immunosuppressive agent.

The occurrence of any complication is a distressing and unwanted event. The current status and future trends in the diagnosis and treatment of lung transplantation complications presented in this chapter provide a brighter scenario for future recipients. However with the present rate of organ referrals, the number of recipients that might benefit from these various advances will be limited.

CHAPTER 6

LONG-TERM FOLLOWUP AND REHABILITATION OF HEART TRANSPLANT PATIENTS

Sharon A. Hunt

INTRODUCTION

The stated goal of cardiopulmonary transplantation is to prolong patients' lives and to restore these patients to an improved quality of life and enable them to resume family life and occupational pursuits. In the early 1990s, 85-90% of previously moribund heart transplant recipients and 60% of heart-lung recipients survived the first postoperative year, and over 50% of heart recipients survived beyond five years, attesting to the achieved goal of prolongation, or improved quantity of life. Documentation of patients' quality of life postoperatively is much more difficult to establish since the endpoints to be achieved are much less amenable to easy quantitation than are endpoints such as survival. This chapter will try to review what has been previously documented as far as function and rehabilitation after transplantation as well as discuss the nature of ongoing impediments to rehabilitation for transplant recipients and prospects for improvements in the future, in terms of both medical and societal impediments.

PHYSIOLOGIC REHABILITATION

Several studies in the early years of cardiac transplantation documented that the denervated heart relied on atypical adaptive mechanisms but had normal resting hemodynamics and a sustained capacity to support normal physical activity.[1,2] The "atypical" adaptive mechanisms had to do mainly with the lack of immediate response of heart rate to stimuli such as exercise which would "ordinarily" lead to increased heart rate through autonomic stimulation of positive chronotropic responses. Without such input the denervated heart was seen to revert automatically to reliance on the intrinsic Frank-Starling mechanism and augment stroke volume in response to increased filling pressures, seen as a prompt increase in LVEDP with exercise. Cardiac index increase per 100 ml/min increase in oxygen uptake ("exercise factor") was normal in the eight patients studied in the first paper published in 1972. With the resurgence of cardiac transplantation in the 1980s, a number of other centers re-documented these findings and additionally noted the new finding of a high prevalence of systemic hypertension in cyclosporine-treated patients.[3,4,5,6] The Pittsburgh group[4] noted a "relatively high" incidence of mild-to-moderate hemodynamic abnormalities at rest at one year postoperatively, the majority of which had normalized or improved by two years postoperatively. Reliance on the Frank-Starling mechanism was demonstrated more elegantly by the London (Ontario) Canada group using radionuclide angiography to compare responses in stroke volume to exercise in transplant versus control groups.[7] They demonstrated that in early exercise, the transplant group had an overall 20% increase in stroke volume as compared to an only slight (3%) increase seen in normal, innervated subjects, and this was associated with the expected slow rate of rise of heart rate in the transplant recipients. Another study from St. Louis confirmed the same physiology but noted some negative correlation between exercise capacity in the early (1 to 3 months) postoperative period and the patient's age and length of hospital stay.[8] By 6 to 12 months postoperative peak exercise capacity correlated mainly with the number of rejection episodes during the first six months, and exercise capacity increased markedly to or toward normal. Another study using radionuclide ventriculography in 28 clinically stable patients early and late after transplantation demonstrated normal to mildly abnormal systolic function and normal diastolic filling properties (measured as peak diastolic filling rate).[9]

Overall, these studies confirm the relatively normal functional capacity of the transplanted heart and correlate nicely with the clinically observed return of patients to routine physical activities. It has been shown by the UCLA group that aggressive, tailored medical therapy for patients with severe heart failure who can be stabilized can result in similar improvement in exercise capacity (although with no change in ejection fraction) at six months of therapy as compared to patients six months post-transplant.[10] It is doubtful, however, that the overall prognosis in such medically-treated patients is changed.

It seems unlikely that future advances can improve upon the already-normal physiologic capabilities of the transplanted heart. Reinnervation, if it occurred or were somehow induced, would simply change the nature of the heart's physiologic adaptive mechanisms, but would not be likely to materially improve upon overall function.

FUNCTIONAL REHABILITATION

While hemodynamic functional indices are fairly straightforward to measure, assessment of quality of life for transplant recipients is more difficult. The first two papers to address this issue described 16 of 25 (64%)[11] and later 51 of 69 (74%)[12] who returned to their previous occupation or activities. Occupations returned to included mechanic, salesman, executive, musician, winemaker, dentist, podiatrist, and professional athlete as well as a number who resumed their interrupted education as students. In the data in these articles an additional four of the 25 (16%)[11] and 11 of the 69 (16%) were in Functional Class I cardiac status, but "voluntarily" retired. Given the structure of the U.S. disability system and its rules, as well as the difficulty encountered by transplant recipients in securing employment, it is not clear how "voluntary" most of these retirements have been. A later study in 1981 from the same group assessed the quality of cardiac function and lifestyle of 25 patients who survived five or more years after transplantation.[13] In this group the average survival period was 6.5 years (range 5.0-10.5 years), and the group provided a total of 167.75 patient-years to follow-up. Defining rehabilitation as ability to perform tasks of interest, work, and have an overall sense of well-being, 143.5 (86%) of these patient years qualified as rehabilitated. This group had less than one non-routine hospitalization per year and 64% were employed, similar to the employment incidence reported after coronary bypass grafting in those days.

In a questionnaire investigation of 23 patients who were under age 30 at the time of transplant, the same group tabulated patient responses to questions regarding health and general fitness, daily living activity restrictions, transportation restrictions, work and school, and marital and life satisfaction.[14] The responses suggested that cardiac transplantation provided genuine rehabilitation in the majority of patients. Of interest, 65% of these patients considered their health to be better than or about the same as that of most people their own age. All 23 patients were able to walk at least one mile, and 70% could walk three miles or more. Eighty-seven percent could do heavy domestic chores such as shovelling snow or cleaning windows. 91% drove their cars, and 87% considered themselves free to come and go as they wanted. Regardless of whether they were in fact gainfully employed, no patient considered him/herself unable to work. Marital satisfaction and sexual function were likewise good for the majority of patients. Overall, 57% were very satisfied with their life after transplantation, 30% were moderately satisfied, 13% were slightly satisfied and none were dissatisfied. 96% stated that they would make the same decision regarding transplantation if they had it to do over.

Another questionnaire study from the Cambridge group used the Nottingham Health Profile (NHP) to provide a quantitative assessment of patient perception of well-being before and at various intervals after heart transplantation.[15] This profile asks patients to respond to direct statements regarding six aspects of their health status: physical mobility, pain, sleep, energy, social isolation, and emotional reactions. In their group of 29 patients responding serially at three months, one year, and two years post-transplant, the scores in all areas fell from severely abnormal preoperatively to those of people in an essentially normal state of health by three months, with stable or improving scores out to two years. The Harefield group used the same NHP questionnaire to assess their 25 patients over the age of 60 at transplant; even

in this older group the results are quite similar, with all patients scoring in the normal self-perception range by six months postop.[16]

In a very interesting study Roger Evans has summarized both objective and subjective indicators of quality of life comparing heart transplant recipients with kidney transplant recipients and dialysis patients and with the general population.[17] In this comparison heart and kidney recipients enjoy a similar quality of life which is not different from the general population and quite superior to that of dialysis patients. Some representative data from this study are shown in Figure 1 and Figure 2.

CONCLUSION

Thus, review of the existing published data suggests that the majority of recipients of heart transplants are in fact fully functional and "well" in both objective and subjective senses. Disability, when it exists, is not commonly due to cardiac causes but usually relates to sequellae of the immunosuppressive regimen such as opportunistic infections or steroid side effects. Two increasingly important and related issues in these patients, however, frequently impact greatly on their postoperative quality of life. These issues are their employability and their insurability. Unless a patient is self-employed or on medical leave from a job being held open for him or her, finding a job after a heart or heart-lung transplant can be quite difficult. Many employers do not want to hire a person with what they view as serious health problems and the potential for unpredictable and possibly lengthy hospitalizations or time off the job. Also, health insurance, if not continued from the preoperative period, is virtually unavailable through any but the largest employers. These factors, which are societal rather than medical, can clearly make what would otherwise be an excellent quality of life socioeconomically most difficult for many patients. They are issues which will need to be addressed more actively in our society over the coming years as increasing numbers of transplant recipients each year return to a functional life and seek to exercise that function in society.

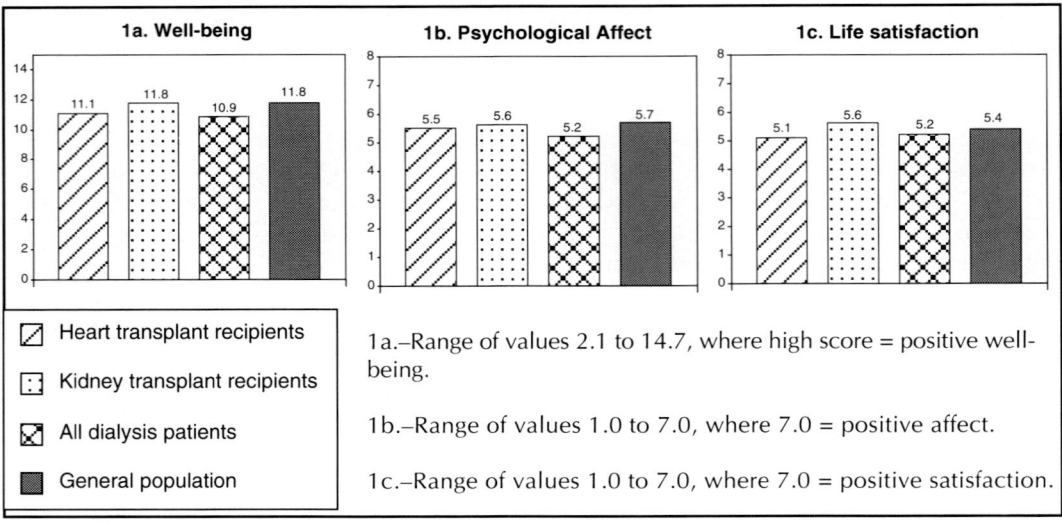

Fig. 1. Subjective indicators of quality of life.[17]

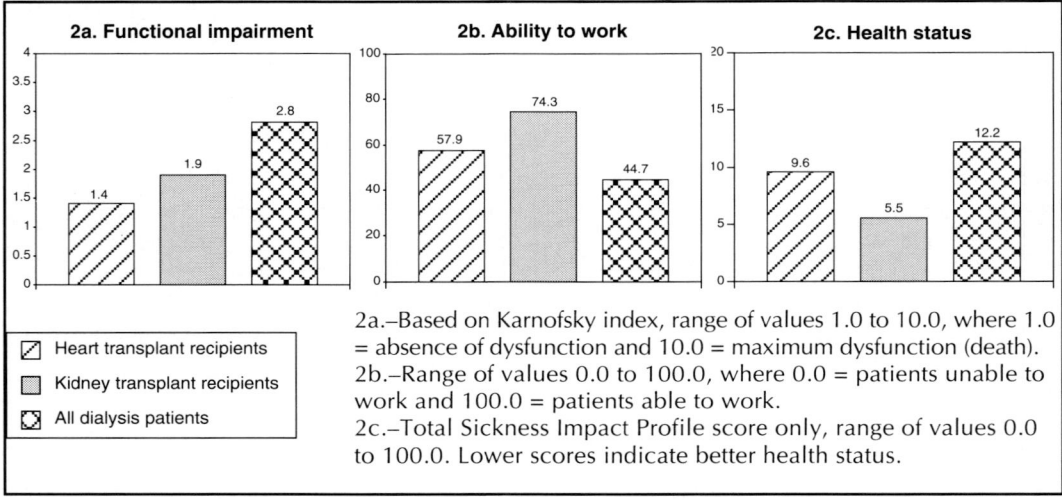

Fig. 2. Objective indicators of quality of life.[17]

THE FUTURE

Future developments in both the world of medicine and in the realm of health care delivery may well impact favorably upon the functional rehabilitation of cardiopulmonary allograft recipients. Medical advances can be expected to provide improved and less toxic modalities of immunosuppression and thus lead to a lessening of the rates of postoperative complications and rehospitalizations. This in turn could lead to a more favorable view of allograft recipients in the job market and workplace. Introduction of a new, centralized, potentially government-supported method of health-care delivery could remove the financial onus currently inherent in hiring a transplant recipient or in the recipient providing his/her own health care coverage. In this projected more ideal world, transplant recipients will be much more truly rehabilitated in the sense of their being returned from the brink of death due to a fatal illness to being self-sufficient and productive members of society.

REFERENCES

1. Stinson EB, Griepp RB, Schroeder JS et al. Hemodynamic observations one and two years after cardiac transplantation in man. Circulation 1972; 45:1183-94.

2. Campeau L, Pospisil L, Groudin P et al. Cardiac catheterization findings at rest and after exercise in patients following cardiac transplantation. Amer J Cardiol 1970; 25:523-28.

3. Pflugfelder PW, McKenzie FN, Kostuk WJ. Hemodynamic profiles at rest and during supine exercise after orthotopic cardiac transplantation. Amer J Cardiol 1988; 61:1328-33.

4. Greenberg ML, Uretsky BF, Reddy S et al. Long-term hemodynamic follow-up of cardiac transplant patients treated with cyclosporine and prednisone. Circulation 1985; 71:487-494.

5. Corcos T, Tamburino C, Leger P et al. Early and late hemodynamic evaluation after cardiac transplantation: A study of 28 cases. JACC 1988; 11:264-69, 1988.

6. Degre SG, Niset GL, De Smet JM et al. Cardiorespiratory response to early exercise testing after orthotopic cardiac transplantation. Amer J Cardiol 1987; 60:926-28.

7. Pflugfelder PW, Purves PD, McKenzie FN, Kostuk WJ. Cardiac dynamics during supine exercise in cyclosporine-treated orthotopic heart transplant recipients: Assessment by radionuclide angiography. JACC 1987; 10:336-41.

8. Labovitz AJ, Drimmer AM, McBride LR et al. Exercise capacity during the first year after cardiac transplantation. Amer J Cardiol 1989; 64:642-45.

9. Verani MS, George SE, Leon CA et al. Systolic and diastolic ventricular performance at rest and during exercise in heart transplant recipients. J Heart Transpl 1987; 7:145-51.

10. Stevenson LW, Sietsema K, Tillisch JH et al. Exercise capacity for survivors of cardiac transplantation or sustained medical therapy for stable heart failure. Circulation 1990; 81:78-85.

11. Graham AF, Schroeder JS, Griepp RB et al. Does cardiac transplantation significantly prolong life and improve its quality? Circulation 1973; 47-48 (Suppl III):III 116-19.

12. Hunt SA, Rider AK, Stinson EB et al. Does cardiac transplantation prolong life and improve its quality? An updated report. Circulation 1976; 54 (Suppl III):III 56-60.

13. Gaudiani VA, Stinson EB, Alderman E et al. Long-term survival and function after cardiac transplantation. Ann Surgery 1981; 194:381-85.

14. Samuellson RG, Hunt SA, Schroeder JS. Functional and social rehabilitation of heart transplant recipients under age thirty. SC and J Thor Cardiovasc Surg 1984; 18:97-103.

15. Hakim M, Spieglehalter D, Elglish TAH et al. Cardiac transplantation with cyclosporine and steroids: Medium and long-term results. Transpl Proc 1988; 20:327-332.

16. Aravot DJ, Banner NR, Khagani A et al. Cardiac transplantation in the seventh decade of life. Amer J Cardiol 1989; 63:90-93.

17. Evans RW. Cost-effectiveness analysis of transplantation. Surg Clin of N Amer 1986; 66:603-16.

CHAPTER 7

LONG-TERM HISTOLOGIC CHANGES IN HEART AND HEART-LUNG ALLOGRAFT RECIPIENTS

Tony R. Zerbe

INTRODUCTION

Cardiac transplantation is now an effective and accepted therapy for end-stage cardiac failure. In the last decade, transplant centers performed over 10,000 cardiac replacements.[1] There is no doubt that this treatment alternative will continue to be available into the next century. While heart-lung and lung transplantations are still emerging as experimental therapies, short-term results are steadily improving. Over 250[2] heart-lung and lung transplants have been performed ensuring that this therapy also will continue to be available.

The one-year survival rate for cardiac transplant recipients has neared the 90% level because of the introduction of the specific immunosuppressive agent cyclosporine and improvements in medical care. Survival rates are considerably less for the complete heart-lung experience, but recent experience shows improvement. When offering such life-saving therapies, knowledge of the one-year survival may not be enough. We have estimated the half-life for the heart and heart-lung recipients in the cyclosporine era using the approach of Terasaki.[3] The half-lives are 7.6 and 7.4 years respectively. (Fig.1) These half-lives are about that seen for the cadaveric renal allograft. This increase in half-life represents an improvement compared to experience with azathioprine and steroids. The focus of attention in the coming decade will be on the reduction of the rate of recipient attrition. Causes for this attrition include infection, malignancy, and chronic graft failure. This chapter will address the observed long term changes that may lead to chronic graft failure.

Pathologists recognize many long-term degenerative structural changes in the allograft heart and lung. The problem is whether these degenerative changes represent a result of an immune response to the foreign tissue (chronic rejection) or follow inflammatory processes associated with transplantation. The result may be the same,

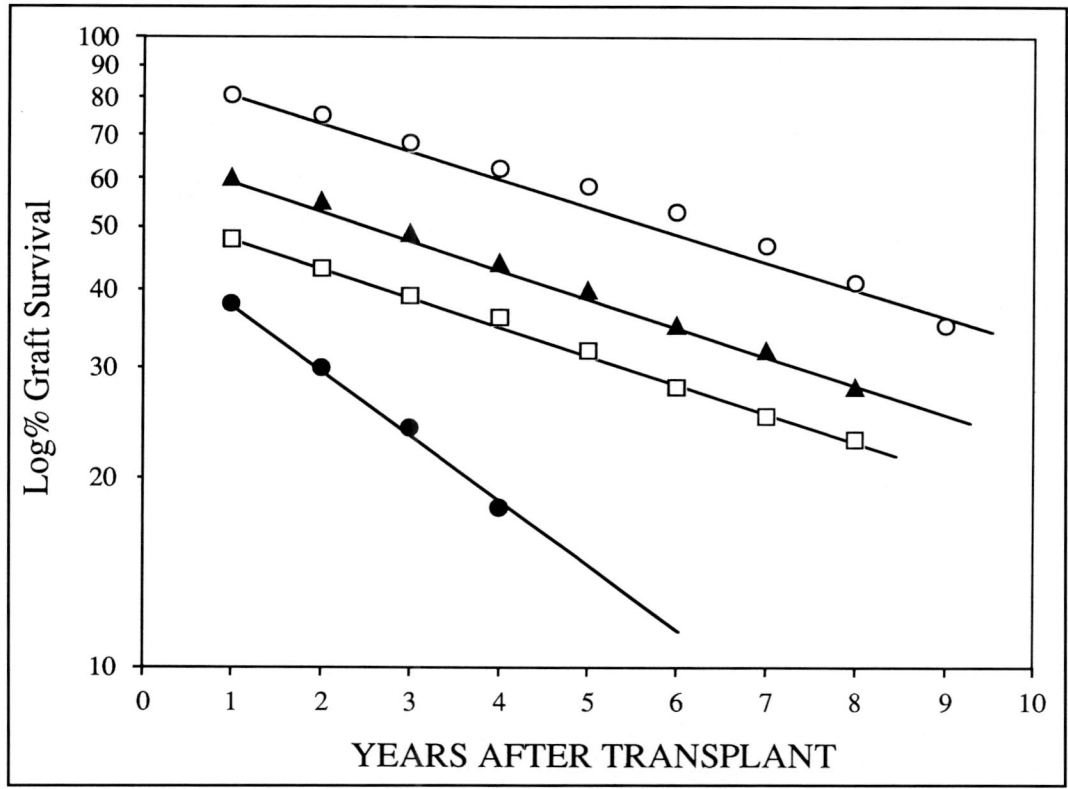

Fig. 1. Long term recipient survival for cardiac allograft experience for several treatment eras. The loss rate is linear for each recipient category: total cardiac allograft experience with cyclosporine at PUH (○), total heart-lung experience with cyclosporine at PUH (▲), cardiac allograft experience with conventional immunosuppression with RATG*(□), cardiac allograft experience with conventional immunosuppression alone* (●). Half-life for conventional immunosuppression alone is 3.7 years. All others experience half-lives of about 7.5 years.* [from Modry et al.]

but identifying this difference is crucial and will influence our approach to this problem.

We will discuss the experience with the heart and the heart-lung transplant separately. Although it is likely that there are many underlying similarities of pathogenetic mechanisms, the morphologic manifestations are different and justify this approach.

LONG TERM CHANGES IN THE ALLOGRAFT HEART

NONCORONARY PATHOLOGY

The transplant community focuses much attention on the coronary arteries of the allograft. There are, in fact, many other morphologic changes seen in long term heart grafts. These may include one or more of the following: pericardial fibrosis, myopathic changes, endocardial and interstitial fibrosis, endocardial lymphocytic infiltrates, and recurrent primary disease. We do not include the cardiac valves in this list. The valves have drawn little comment in the literature. We recognize no macroscopic alterations in these structures in our autopsy series.

Pericardial Fibrosis

Pericardial fibrosis is a universal finding in grafts that survive the immediate postoperative period. Severe pericardial fibrosis leads to functional compromise. This is an infrequent finding in our autopsy experience, occurring in less than 2% of all cases.

Myopathy

In our experience, myocyte changes noted

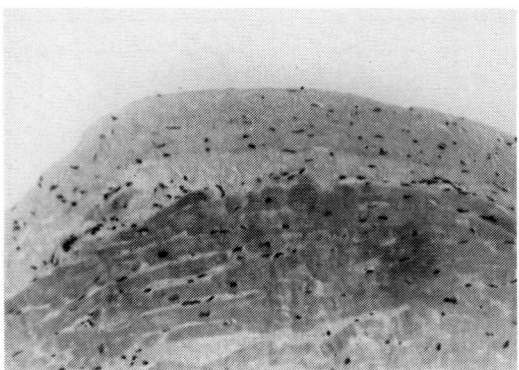

Fig. 2. H & E section of endomyocardial biopsy showing thickening of the endocardial layer. Normally the endocardium consists of a single layer of endothelium and a few layers of fibroblasts and fibrous connective tissue. A slight interstitial fibrosis is present in this sample as well.

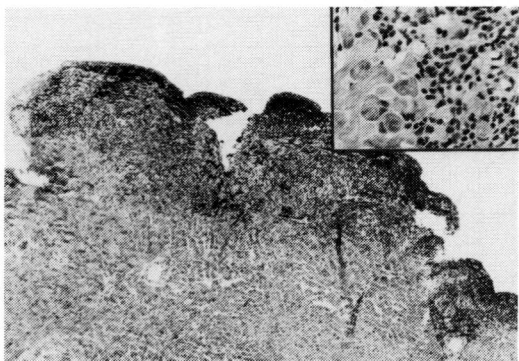

Fig. 3. H & E section of endomyocardial biopsy showing a localized thickening of the endocardial layer by an infiltrate of small mononuclear cells. A large aggregate contains numerous small vessels. At the base of the aggregate, lymphocytes stream down into the underlying muscle (inset).

in the biopsies of the right ventricle are similar to those seen in cardiomyopathies. Most recipients have grafts that show this change. This is not the case for most heart-lung recipients.

At autopsy, the allograft usually shows a marked increase in muscle mass, with both right and left ventricular hypertrophy. The systemic hypertension associated with cyclosporine therapy certainly would not explain the right ventricular changes. Pulmonary hypertension is not a recognized problem in this population. Chronic ischemia from coronary narrowing is another readily available but as yet untested hypothesis. Imakita suggests this hypertrophy follows from effects of preservation.[4]

When seen, the degree of myocyte hypertrophy is so striking that it suggests there may be some primary myocyte dysfunction occurring as well. Recent animal studies show inflammatory cytokine effects on myocyte function through the inhibition of membrane receptor activity.[5] This non-lethal effect upon the myocyte could explain the dysfunction seen in hearts with so little evidence of myocyte necrosis. This remains an incompletely addressed area.

Endocardial and Interstitial Fibrosis

Endocardial and interstitial fibrosis is an almost universal finding in the biopsy from the allograft heart after six months. (Fig. 2) Kendall et al show that the extent of this

fibrosis correlates with cardiac dysfunction.[6] Whether the fibrosis is a result of healed rejection, ischemia from coronary artery disease, drug effect or other injury is not clear. Recent studies show that some of this fibrosis may be a result of injury occurring during preservation.[7] That the harvest or preservation injury may cause a late fibrotic reaction is a very important observation. We must take this into account when examining coronary disease and drug effects.

We recognize structural changes due to cyclosporine toxicity in the allograft kidney and also in the native kidneys of recipients of other types of organ grafts.[8,9] We have not found reports of interstitial fibrosis or vessel wall deposits occurring in the native hearts or lungs of renal or hepatic graft recipients. It is still unclear whether there are specific structural changes in the allograft heart related to cyclosporine.[10] We have offered other possible explanations for the interstitial fibrosis above. This question remains open.

Endocardial Lymphocytic Infiltrates

Endocardial lymphocytic infiltrates are a unique lesion which appear only in the allograft heart. (Fig. 3) Billingham reports rarely seeing this lesion in the allograft before the introduction of cyclosporine.[11] She identified this lesion in about 9% of the biopsies in which cyclosporine is used. In our experience with cyclosporine, these lesions

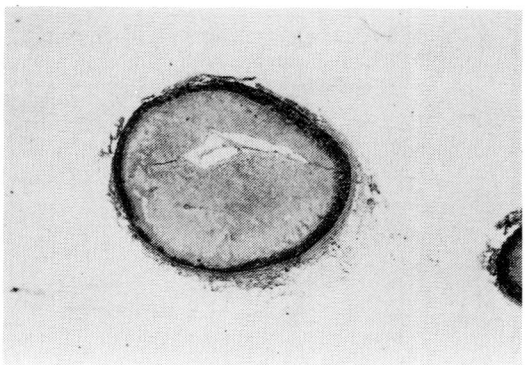

Fig. 4. H & E section of an epicardial coronary vesel from an allograft heart. The lumen is concentrically narrowed by a proliferation of smooth muscle cells. The elastic lamina and media are generally intact. Focal breakdown of the intima with cholesterol is noted forming an atheroma.

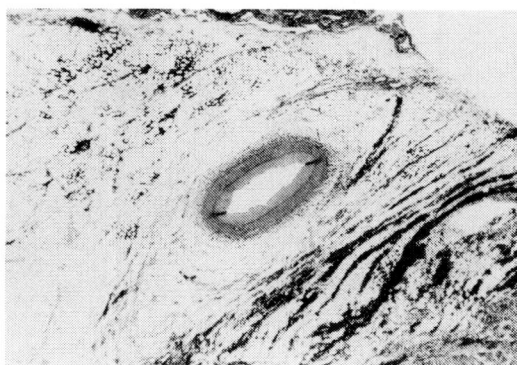

Fig. 5. H & E section of an epicardial coronary vessel from an allograft heart that failed in less than four days. Note the concentric intima with intact elastic lamina.

were present in 5.4% of biopsies. In a smaller series with FK506, these lesions were present in only 1.2% of biopsies. This is a reduction when compared to cyclosporine.

The explanations offered for endocardial lymphocytic infiltrates have included a form of post-transplant immunoproliferative disorder[12] or peculiar response to the endocardium.[13] We have shown these infiltrates correlate with a history of cellular rejection and with angiogram evidence of coronary disease.[14] We support the belief that these infiltrates represent a form of endothelial inflammation that reflects inflammation in the coronary vessels. Our work did not identify any Epstein-Barr viral genome in a sample of our examples of this unique infiltrate.

Recurrent Disease

Valantine reported the only recurrence of a primary disease thus far, and that is systemic amyloidosis.[15] Our patients who have died from problems related to systemic amyloidosis, have shown severe cardiac allograft amyloid. Although amyloidosis is an immune system dysfunction, the recurrences seen are not likely to represent a chronic inflammatory response to the graft.

CORONARY PATHOLOGY

The chronic changes seen in the epicardial coronaries have attracted the most attention

of all the long-term changes noted in the allograft heart. In the early years of cardiac transplantation essentially all patients developed a rapidly progressive vessel narrowing termed post-transplant arteriopathy.[16,17] The underlying mechanism remains undefined, but a widely held view is that the arteriopathy represents chronic rejection.

Diagnostic Features

Billingham recently reviewed the morphologic features of this form of arteriopathy.[11,18] Diffuse and concentric intimal hyperplasia of the myofibroblast (Fig. 4) are the hallmarks of this form of vascular disease. There may be a marked lymphocytic inflammatory infiltrate of the intima. The lack of disruption of the elastic lamina is another feature used to discriminate from native vessel disease.

Specificity

We have not seen results that address how specific these features are in distinguishing arteriopathy from native coronary disease. We reviewed the coronary vessels from the allografts that failed in the immediate postoperative period, and identified intimal hyperplasia in the epicardial coronaries of these donor organs. (Fig. 5) Our interpretation is that this must represent the early stages of native atherosclerosis. Occasional coronary vessels from native organs also exhibit features similar to those of post-transplant arteriopathy. (Fig. 6) Physical injury can cause such concentric intimal hyperplasia.[19]

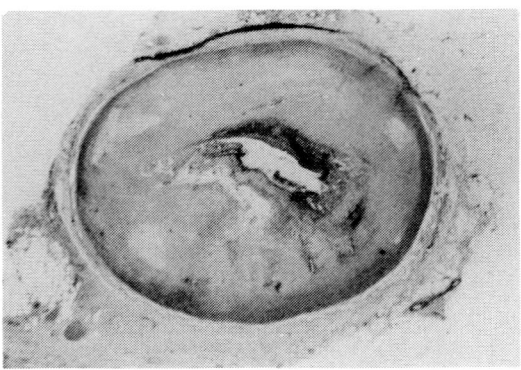

Fig. 6. H & E section of an epicardial coronary vessel from a native heart with ischemic heart disease. The section shows concentric intimal thickening focal atheroma. In this vessel the media and elastic lamina show some areas of damage. The features are quite similar to those seen in Figure 4.

The luminal narrowing seen in this study of the donor organs ranged from 0 to 72% (mean 30%). (Fig. 7) This finding suggests that some donor organs have early changes of atherosclerosis at the time of transplant, while others may have fairly advanced disease. This advanced disease may appear on the coronary angiogram after transplantation. We do not yet know the effect of preservation, drug therapy, or rejection on the early lesions.

We do not know the exact incidence of post-transplant arteriopathy, since diagnosis relies on coronary angiography. This method is itself subject to problems in identification of coronary vessel narrowing.[20] This method cannot identify the important features for distinguishing native disease from post-transplant arteriopathy. Information to date suggests that upwards of 50% of recipients have angiogram identifiable disease by the fifth year following the transplant.[21] Thrombotic compromise can result is myocardial infarct. (Fig. 8)

POTENTIAL MECHANISMS

Within the past decade several studies have identified risk factors for this process. As with native atherosclerosis these studies have focused upon the patients lipid status, history of viral infection, and allograft immune response as a triggering or perpetuating injury.

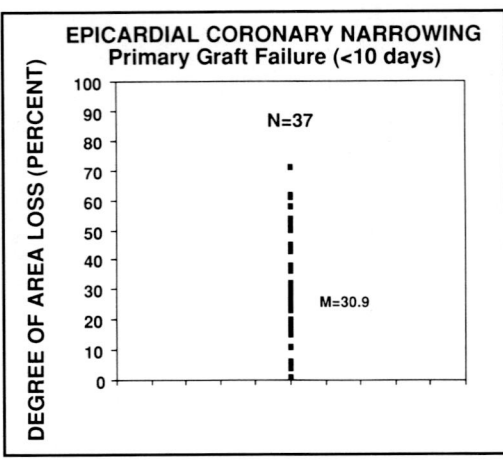

Fig. 7. This graph depicts the range of luminal narrowing measured from 37 cardiac grafts that failed within the first 10 days. The narrowing is determined by planimetry from photomicrographs of sections of epicardial coronary vessels. The range is from 0% to 72% with a mean luminal narrowing of 30%.

Lipid Status

Gao et al[22] and Winters[23] et al reported an association with post-transplant lipid levels and body mass and the development of the disease. Changing the sources of dietary lipid content reduces vessel narrowing. This occurs in the allograft animal when compared to immunosuppressive agents alone or other anti-inflammatory agents.[24] Hyperlipidemia is a complication of current immunosuppressive drug regimens. FK506 does not have this

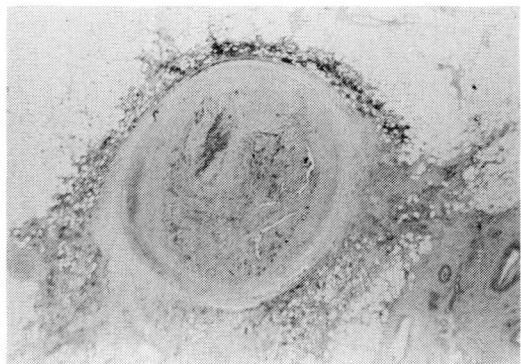

Fig. 8. H & E section of a right coronary vessel from an allograft with chronic failure. This section shows complete occlusion of the lumen by organizing thrombus. The adventitia shows inflammation and fibrosis. No proliferation of the intima is observed.

association. We find it difficult to incorporate the lipid association into a hypothesis of chronic rejection due in part to the identical association with native atherosclerosis.

Viral Infection

Grattan et al[25] showed that severe arteriopathy arises earlier in patients who have infection by cytomegalovirus (CMV) infection. In his study, he defined severe arteriopathy as 70% or greater narrowing. His CMV positive group experienced more episodes of rejection than the CMV negative group. He offered several explanations involving direct or indirect action of CMV to explain this association. The direct mechanisms include viral mediation of endothelial injury or intimal hyperplasia. The indirect mechanisms include antibody mediated injury and induction of new or increased levels of cell antigens.

Support for the direct mechanisms would come with the demonstration of viral antigen or genome in the lesions. Hruban [26] reported identification of viral genome in the vessels of allograft hearts. We see viral genome for the herpes viruses, simplex or cytomegalic, in less than 2% of coronary vessels studied at autopsy. We used both immunohistochemistry and insitu methods. Others have identified viral material in native vessels with these techniques.[27] Recent work shows polymerase chain reaction (PCR) can identify viral genome in vascular tissue when other methods fail.[28] Application of such methods to transplant arteriopathy will certainly lay this question of viral material in the vessel to rest.

The indirect action of the virus in inciting an inflammatory response is more difficult to decipher and to separate from the action of rejection. The response to CMV is complex in the normal host and the addition of immunosuppressive agents further confounds the response. The natural immunity conveyed by cytotoxic cells can also lead to severe immunopathogenic injury. Several laboratories are defining the action of cytotoxic cells and the inflammatory cytokines such as interferon gamma and tumor necrosis factor on endothelial cells.[29,30] The data presented by Grattan[25] and others[31] shows that CMV may incite an allograft specific immune

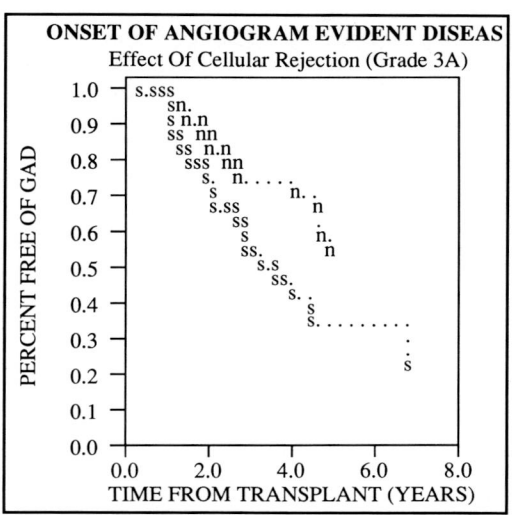

Fig. 9. This graph shows the results of a life table analysis which compared two groups of cardiac allograft recipients. One group designated by the (s) did experience an episode of moderate cellular rejection (grade 3A or greater). The second group designated by the (n) did not experience an episode of rejection. The analysis compared the time of detection of coronary disease by angiogram. The y axis is the percent of each group free of coronary disease, the x axis is the time from transplant in years. The incidence of coronary disease and time to onset are different between the two groups (p<.01). [Reprinted with permission from Zerbe T. Graft atherosclerosis: Effects of cellular rejection and human lymphocyte antigen, J Heart and Lung Transp 1992; 11:104. Copyright Mosby-Year Book, Inc.]

response that breaks through treatment. Grattan's report did not address the participation of rejection in coronary arteriopathy for the CMV negative group.

Rejection

Uretsky reported an association of cellular rejection and vessel disease.[21] He did not separate control for the occurrence of CMV infection. We have extended this work to show a very strong association with the presentation of angiogram-evident coronary disease and acute cellular rejection. (Fig. 9) Multivariant analysis to isolate effects of lipid level or infection status is yet to be completed.

Hruban,[32] Herskowitz,[33] Palmer,[34] Salomon[35] and our group[36] have reported the presence of a lymphocytic intimitis in the coronary ves-

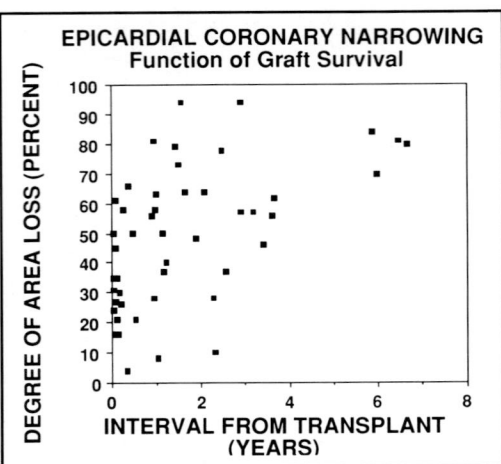

Fig. 10. This graph shows the results of direct measurement of coronary vessel narrowing plotted against the interval from transplant in years. The narrowing is determined by planimetry from photomicrographs of sections of epicardial coronary vessels. The narrowing ranged from 3% to over 90%. Note there is considerable variation, but there is a trend to increase narrowing with interval from transplant.

sels of some grafts at autopsy. Kaufman has isolated alloreactive lymphocytes from all samples of coronary vessels after transplantation.[37] These findings say there is a cellular reaction present in the coronary. This occurs without cellular rejection in the myocardium. We must now focus on identifying the target of this coronary lymphocytic reaction. It is possible that the enhanced expression of HLA antigens on the endothelium causes this infiltrate.

Examination of coronary vessel sections taken at autopsy shows that all allograft organs have some degree of coronary narrowing. (Fig. 10) In all but a few of our cases the luminal narrowing is concentric with involvement of penetrating vessels. We used linear regression to assess the degree of luminal narrowing in this series. (Fig. 11) Thus far the analysis has identified only duration from transplant and the occurrence of moderate rejection as predictive variables. These results show that any episode of moderate rejection adds only a relatively small increment of narrowing (10%) to the process. The equation predicts a luminal narrowing of 7% to 8% occurs per year. We do not now have the numbers of cases required to further dissect the causes of this narrowing.

Support for a humoral mechanism comes from the work of Hess,[38] Reemstra[39] and others. Their investigations show that the presence of cytotoxic antibodies to lymphocytes reduces cardiac recipient survival. Allograft coronary disease is more frequent in the group with such antibodies. This supports the work of Minick[40] and Laden[41] in animals. There are reports of humoral components present in the coronary vessels.[34] These reports do not explain the presence of a cellular infiltrate in

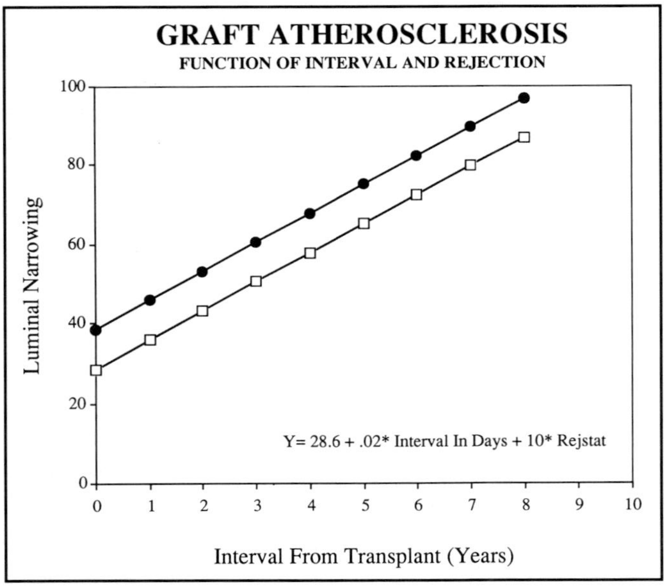

GRAFT ATHEROSCLEROSIS
FUNCTION OF INTERVAL AND REJECTION

Y= 28.6 + .02* Interval In Days + 10* Rejstat

Interval From Transplant (Years)

Luminal Narrowing

Fig. 11. This graph shows a plot of the linear equation derived from a regression analysis of the luminal narrowing data depicted in Figure 10. The two lines represent recipients who have experienced an episode of rejection (●) and recipients who have not experienced an episode of rejection (□). Experiencing cellular rejection adds a constant increment of narrowing of 10% to luminal narrowing that progressively increases with time. Note the y intercept (29%), narrowing at time of transplant, is similar to that determined from the study of the grafts with early failure (30%).

the lesion, unless this reaction is a type of antibody dependent cytotoxic process. This is an avenue of injury that has not received attention.

These findings offer fairly strong support that an alloimmune reaction is the culprit in allograft coronary atherosclerosis. However, native atherosclerosis contains a similar less intense lymphocytic infiltrate.[42] The location of infiltrate in native disease is at the interface of the sclerotic plaque and the media. Patients with native atherosclerosis also exhibit a humoral response to several antigens.[43,44] Other potential causes of endothelial injury are present in the allograft situation. The global ischemia of preservation may cause a sublethal endothelial injury very similar to that induced in experimental models. These models use direct mechanical injury to induce intimal hyperplasia.[19] We have mentioned the effect of medication.

LONG-TERM CHANGES IN THE ALLOGRAFT LUNG

The investigators working with the allograft lung are focusing on the occurrence of obliterative bronchiolitis (OB). There are other long-term changes in the lung as well, but none with the clinical results of OB. The other changes described thus far involve the pleura, bronchial cartilage and pulmonary arteries. Investigators are likely to identify additional changes as experience with this allograft and patient survival increases.

The pleura reaction is one of various degrees of fibrosis. The fibrosis rarely will be so extensive as to obliterate the pleural space or restrict lung motion. Minor degrees of pleural reaction, however, can lead to pleural fusion and angiogenesis that can complicate additional surgery.

Yousem recently described a degenerative change of the bronchial cartilage.[45] The patterns of this finding suggested ischemic effect as a result of bronchial artery ligation during transplant. This also may act as an alternative stimulus for bronchial scarring.

The pulmonary artery changes are similar to those seen in the coronary arteries of the allograft heart but they are not obstructive. Tazelarr[2] and Yousem[46] described an active

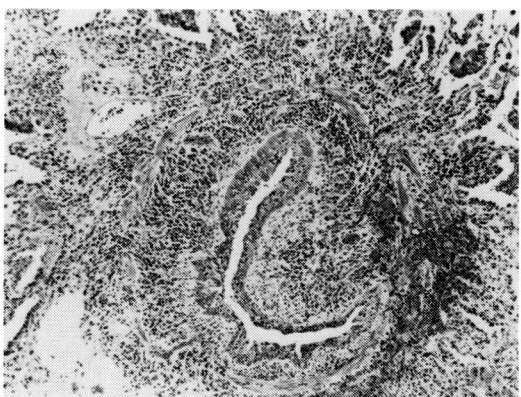

Fig. 12. H & E section of small airway of the allograft lung showing lymphocytic inflammation of the muscularis, submucosa, and epithelium.

intimal inflammation similar to that seen in the allograft coronary disease. They also raised the possibility that pulmonary hypertension may be an eventual result.

Obliterative Bronchiolitis

Obliterative bronchiolitis is a fibrotic process that by definition leads to luminal obliteration of the terminal airways. In this way OB is like allograft coronary disease. The process of OB is exuberant granulation that occurs after inflammation or ulceration of the bronchial epithelium. The granulation can completely resolve, lead to submucosal scars, or result in complete obliteration of the small airway. (Figs. 12-13)

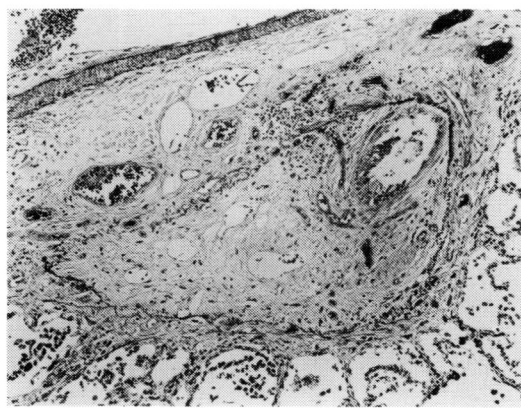

Fig. 13. H & E section of small airway of the allograft lung showing almost complete obliteration of the lumen by fibrous tissue. A bronchial artery is seen nearby that shows some focal intimal proliferation.

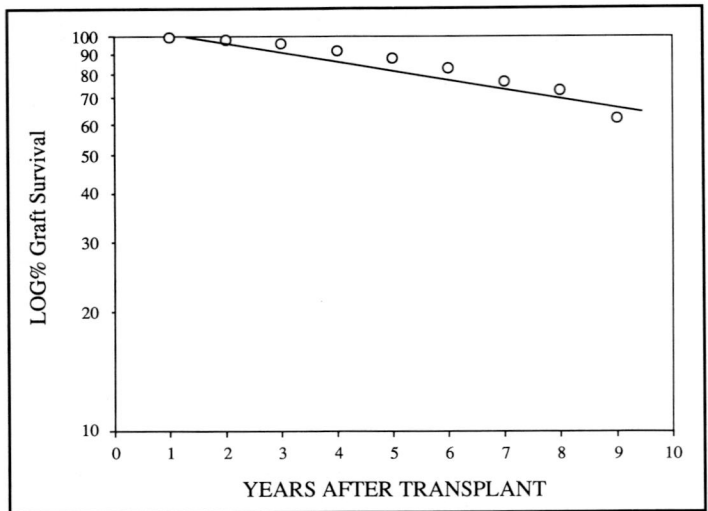

Fig. 14. Long-term recipient survival for cardiac allograft experience with chronic graft failure. The loss rate is linear for this recipient category: total cardiac allograft experience with cyclosporine at PUH (○). Half-life based upon extrapolation of data is 13.5 years.

Obliterative bronchiolitis in the allograft leads to a progressive reduction in lung function. Reports of the incidence in the transplant population vary, depending upon whether the criteria include clinical features alone or biopsy techniques. In general, like coronary arteriopathy, at least 50% of transplant recipients develop this condition.[47]

In the native lung, OB follows infection and some autoimmune diseases. As a result, the studies of OB in the allograft are focused on rejection and infection. The consensus is that bronchiolitis obliterans is one manifestation of chronic rejection in the allograft. The report of Clelland et al[48] suggests that the degree of cellular rejection experienced predicts the onset of obliterative bronchiolitis.

Sampling by transbronchial biopsy and bronchial alveolar lavage has permitted study of the insitu inflammatory response. Zeevi[49] measured the proliferative response and cellular cytotoxic activity of the cells isolated from these samples. This invitro reactivity is a correlate to the development of OB in the allograft. In contrast to several other immunologic lung diseases, OB does not end in diffuse pulmonary fibrosis.

The report of Fend[50] says that OB is more likely to arise in allograft recipients who experience CMV infection. The results at Pittsburgh support this postinfection association.[47] This is analogous to the reports on allograft coronary disease.

Response to Treatment

Some investigators believe that these chronic graft changes are due to indolent rejection. They say that more specific immunosuppressive agents or better matching for transplantation antigens will reduce both the heart and lung graft loss.[51] It is not clear that this will be the case.

Returning to Figure 1, the survival data says that the rate of patient attrition is similar in the heart and heart-lung recipients. It also shows that the rate of loss is not different between cyclosporine and conventional therapy which includes antithymocyte globulin.[52] This is the case with the renal allograft as well.[3]

We cannot directly equate heart and heart-lung survival with chronic graft failure. In contrast to the majority of renal allograft loss, heart and heart-lung recipient loss is due to many other causes. To determine the cardiac graft half-life requires identifying those graft losses in which chronic degenerative changes have played a major role. This occurs in roughly one-third of all deaths. We see a similar rate in the heart-lung group. Autopsies

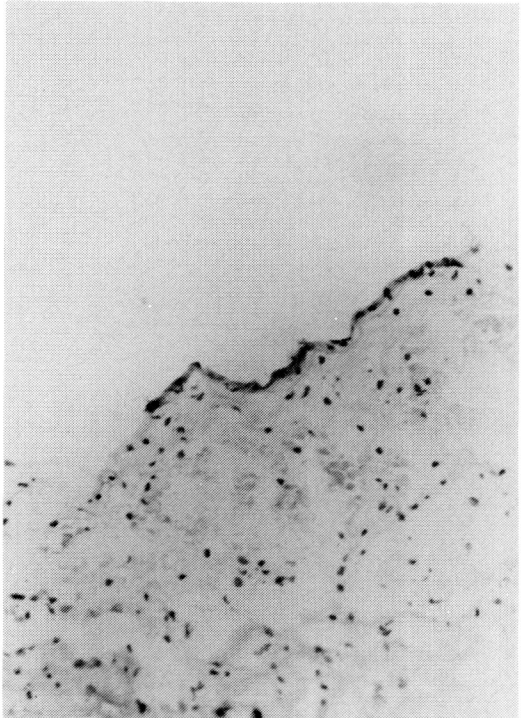

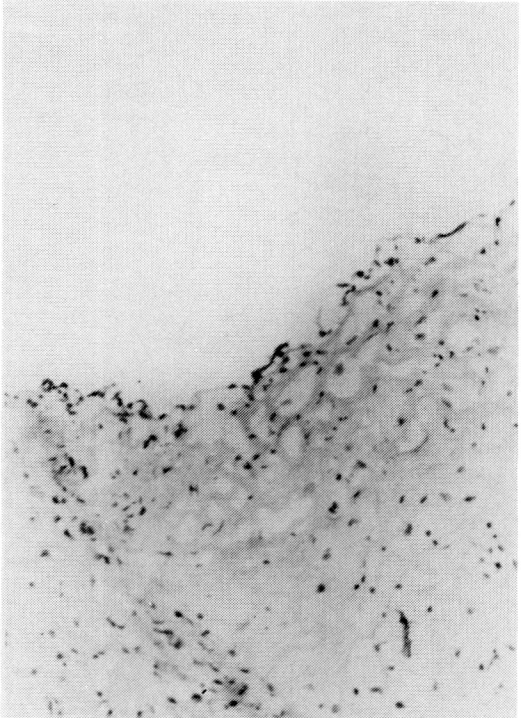

Fig. 15. Frozen section of an epicardial coronary vessel treated with monoclonal antibody to intercellular adhesion molecule (ICAM). Detection of antibody binding was accomplished with antimouse antibody labeled with biotin followed by avidin biotin complex. Development of color reaction was done using aminoethylcarbazole (aec). The endothelium lining the coronary shows uniform expression of ICAM.

Fig. 16. Paraffin section of an epicardial coronary vessel treated with rabbit antibody to endothelial leukocyte adhesion molecule (ELAM). Detection of antibody binding was accomplished with anti-rabbit antibody labeled with biotin followed by avidin biotin complex. Development of color reaction was done using aminoethylcarbazole (aec). The endothelium lining the coronary shows uniform expression of ELAM.

are not available in all deaths. To arrive at a conservative estimate, we assumed that deaths occurring in recipients with coronary disease were due to chronic graft failure.[53] We show the results of this analysis for chronic graft failure in Figure 14. By projecting the survival curve, we arrived at a half-life estimate of 13.5 years. By definition this means only 50% of heart recipients will lose their grafts directly to chronic graft failure in 13.5 years.

We find it interesting that this is double the half-life for cadaveric renal allograft using similar immunosuppressive drugs. This observation suggests to me that the cardiac graft has a survival more like the haplotype mismatched renal allograft. Showing any further effect of therapy or HLA matching will require pooling of results from many centers.

Glanville reports slowing of loss of lung function by changing drug treatment.[54] Presumably, this was through action on OB. Glanville achieved this by replacement of a specific T cell immunosuppressive agent with the less specific action of azathioprine. This is consistent with the observation of Laden[41] in the control of coronary disease. It also suggests either a tissue response outside the influence of cyclosporine (antibody type) or that cyclosporine has an unrecognized toxicity that affects only transplanted organs.[55]

These observations suggest that it may be necessary to continue investigation of the fibrotic process in these two conditions to identify regulatory states. At the least, further investigation can only improve our understanding of this process in the native organ.

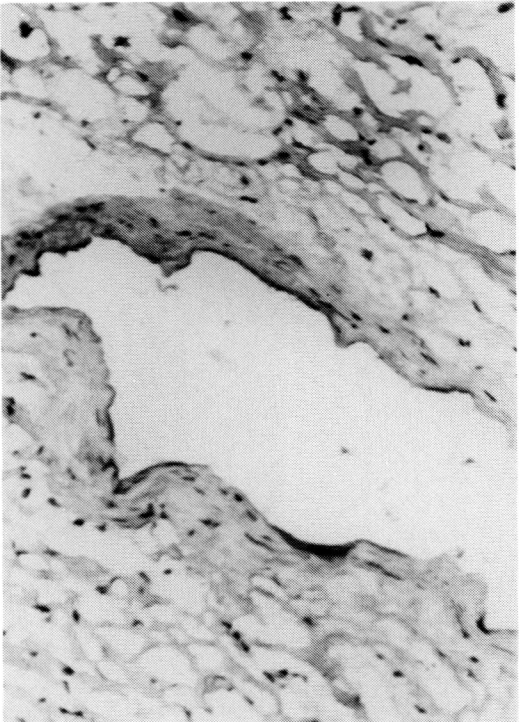

Fig. 17. Frozen section of a myocardium treated with mouse antibody to angiotensin converting enzyme (ACE). Detection of antibody binding was accomplished with antimouse antibody labeled with biotin followed by avidin biotin complex. Development of color reaction was done using aminoethylcarbazole (aec). The endothelium lining the myocardial vessels shows uniform expression of ACE.

Future Directions

This parallel trail of evidence has developed for bronchiolitis obliterans and coronary arteriopathy. The evidence strongly suggests these two problems may be different manifestations of a similar underlying mechanism. Reconciling these findings will be the focus of work for this decade and perhaps into the next century.

The experience in clinical transplantation thus far supports that an alloimmune response is sufficient but may not be necessary to induce this fibrotic response. The animal studies of Cramer[56] and Prop[57] show that indolent rejection to major or minor transplantation antigens plays a role in both coronary and bronchial lesions.

To confirm these features as chronic rejection will require showing that recipients without other triggers, including acute rejection, develop either allograft coronary disease or OB. We also need to see whether or not the progress of either disease is affected by the degree of tissue compatibility. To address this question requires a multicenter effort to have enough patients. Further autotransplant studies are needed which condition the autotransplant as donor organs are in practice. This conditioning, combined with exposure to immunosuppressive agents, will show if these factors participate in triggering these fibrotic processes.

The common thread of the coronary and bronchial processes is a fibrotic response. The fibrosis, once started, may become self-perpetuating through interruption of healing. The reports mentioned here show both the coronary and bronchial disease follow infection and rejection. Body lipid levels and hypertension show only an effect on allograft coronary disease. These associations all have in common tissue injury, some through an alloimmune response or possible potentiation of that response. This fits well with the hypothesis for native coronary disease.[58]

The literature shows that de novo expression of several surface molecules follows endothelial injury or stimulation. This ranges from procoagulant to HLA and cell adhesion proteins ICAM and ELAM.[29,30] Duquesnoy recently reviewed the importance of the proteins in the generation of the alloimmune response.[59] He concluded that these proteins are important to the sequestration of activated cells in the allograft. We are currently studying the expression of these proteins in allograft coronary disease. (Figs. 15-16) Bronchial epithelium shows a similar increased expression of surface molecules.[60] The effect of inflammation on class II expression is evidence of this. We expect to find additional responses with the introduction of bronchial epithelial culture.

The allograft coronary disease shows at least one feature that makes it quite different from OB. This feature is the marked smooth muscle proliferation in the intima. We feel that smooth muscle cell proliferation does not occur until after the smooth muscle cells migrate into the intima of the coronary vessel.

Many laboratories are studying the interaction of endothelium and smooth muscle cells. These laboratories use both in vivo and in vitro models. Endothelial cells release several compounds that are locally active.[29,30] The study of smooth muscle cells is complex as these cells undergo a spontaneous change of phenotype in culture. Despite this complexity, several laboratories have identified growth regulatory compounds or systems involved in repair of vascular injury. Two compounds now at the top of the list are basic fibroblast growth factor[61] and transforming growth factor beta.[62] The laboratories involved are studying the regulation of these compounds in the generation of vessel injury.

Following the lead of Powell[19] and Bell[63], our group is studying one endothelial system known to effect vessel response to injury, namely the angiotensin converting enzyme system. This system is present in the vessels of the heart. (Fig. 17) Their invitro experiments show a paracrine regulation of endothelial and smooth muscle cell migration following endothelial conversion of angiotensin I.[19,63] These reports also show that inhibition of angiotensin converting enzyme will stop the migration of smooth muscle into the intima. It is not clear whether angiotensin II is itself chemotactic for smooth muscle, or endothelial cell injury alters the expression or activity of angiotensin converting enzyme. We are pursuing the answers to these questions.

Other investigators identify alternate regulatory systems for endothelium[64] and perhaps for obliterative bronchiolitis a form of pulmonary fibrosis.[65] Additional clinical studies will continue to give insight into these fibrotic processes affecting the allograft heart and lung. The direction for the next decade and perhaps beyond will be toward addressing these questions at the cellular level.

My expectations are that we will continue to see traditional cell culture and animal studies used to study cell regulation. We will see Western and Northern analysis combined with insitu hybridization or immunohistochemistry to further dissect cell responses. My expectations for the next decade are that

we will also see use of two new technologies. These are the technologies of transgenic animals and gene transfer.

Palmiter, Brinster, and Jaenisch recently reviewed the technology of transgenic animals.[66,67] With this technology it is possible to create a stable incorporation of human genes into the genome of animals. Using similar approaches of DNA incorporation, Nabel,[68] Mulligan[69] and others have incorporated human genes into selected animal[70,71] and human[72] tissues for variable periods. Although technical improvements will no doubt continue, we can look forward to using these techniques to address the problem of "Chronic graft loss."

How might we use these new techniques to study allograft loss? Dr. Bach[73] and his group are creating transgenic animals as sources of organs for transplantation. The group intends to overcome the xenograft barrier by incorporating human genes for selected transplantation antigens. In addition it will be possible to ask specific questions about the importance of cell products of endothelium or bronchial epithelium. We can incorporate genes into these tissues programmed to stimulate or block production of selected cell products.[74] With this approach, we may identify the critical factors in the pathogenesis of obliterative arterial and airway disease. Along the way, therapeutic approaches using gene transfer may result.

REFERENCES

1. Kriett JM, Kaye MP. The registry of the international society for heart transplantation; seventh official report: 1990 Heart Transplantation 1990; 9:323-330.
2. Tazelaar HD, Yousem S. The pathology of combined heart-lung transplantation: An autopsy study. Human Pathol 1988; 19:1403-1416.
3. Terasaki PI. Histocompatibility testing in transplantation. Arch Pathol Lab Med 1991; 115:250-254.
4. Imakita M, Tazelaar HD, Rowan RA, Masek MA, Billingham ME. Myocyte hypertrophy in the transplanted heart: A morphometric analysis: Transplantation 1987; 43:839-842.
5. Gulick T, Chung M, Pieper S, Schreiner G, Lange L. Immune cytokine inhibition of beta-adrenergic agonist stimulated cyclic amp generation in cardiac myocytes. Biochem Biophys Commun 1988; 150:1-9
6. Kendall TJ, Winters GL, Radio SJ et al. Concor-

dance of progressions in cardic dysfunction and myo-cardial fibrosis in human heart allografts. Abs International Symposium in Inflammatory Heart Disease July 1988 Snowmass Colo.

7. Pickering JG, Boughner DR. Fibrosis in the transplanted heart and its relation to donor ischemic time. Circulation 1990; 81:949-958.

8. Dische FE, Neuberger J, Keating J et al. Kidney pathology in liver allograft recipients after long term treatment with cyclosporine Lab Invest 1988; 58:395-402.

9. Dieterle A, Gratwohl A, Nizze H et al. Chronic cyclosporine-associated nephrotoxicity in bone marrow transplant recipients. Transplantation 1990; 49:1093-1100.

10. Karch SB, Billingham ME. Cyclosporine induced myocardial fibrosis, a unique controlled case report. Heart Transplantation 1985; 4:210-212

11. Billingham ME. The pathology of organ transplantation. In: Butterworth SG, ed. Cardiac Transplantation. Stoneham: 1990: 133-152.

12. Kemnitz J, Cohnert TR. Lymphoma like lesions in human orthotopic cardiac allografts. Am J Clin Path 1988; 89:430 Abstract.

13. Kottke-Marchant K, Ratliff NB. Endocardial lymphocytic infiltrates in cardiac transplant recipients. Arch Pathol Lab Med 1989; 113:690-698.

14. Zerbe TR. Endocardial lymphocytic infiltrates in cardiac allograft recipients. Abstract 2nd International Conference on Graft Infiltrating Cells 1989 Snowmass, Co.

15. Valantine H, Billingham ME. Recurrence of amyloid in a cardiac allograft four months after transplantation. J Heart Transplant 1989; 4:337-341.

16. Bieber C, Stinson E, Shumway N, Payne R, Kosek J. Cardiac Transplantation in Man. Cardiac Allograft Pathology. Circulation 1970; 41:753-772

17. Baumgartner WA, Reitz BA, Oyer PE, Stinson EB, Shumway NE, Cardiac homotransplantation. Curr Probl Surg 1979; 16:1-61.

18. Billingham ME. Graft coronary disease: The lesions and the patients. Transplant Proc 1989; 21:3665-3666.

19. Powell JS, Clozel JP, Muller RKM et al. Inhibitors of angiotensin-converting enzyme prevent myointimal proliferation after vascular injury. Science 1989; 245:186-188.

20. Paulin S. Assessing the severity of coronary lesions with angiography. Editorial NEJM 1987; 316:1405-6.

21. Uretsky BF, Murali S, Reddy S et al. Development of coronary artery disease in cardiac transplant patients receiveing immunosuppressive therapy with cyclosporing and prednisone. Circulation 1987; 76:827-834.

22. Gao S-Z, Schroeder J, Alderman E, Hunt S et al. Clinical and laboratory correlates of accelerated coronary artery disease in the cardiac transplant patient. Circulation 1987; 76:V56-V61.

23. Winters GL, Kendall TJ, Radio SJ et al. Post transplant obesity and hyperlipidemia: Major predictors

of severity of arteriopathy in failed human heart allograft. Abstract 2nd International Conference on Graft Infiltrating Cells 1989 Snowmass, Co.

24. Sarris GE, Mitchell RS, Billingham ME et al. Inhibition of accelerated cardiac allograft arteriosclerosis by fish oil. J Thorac Cardiovasc Surg 1989; 97:841-855.

25. Grattan MT, Moreno-Cabal CE, Starnes VA et al. Cytomegalovirus infection is associated with cardiac allograft rejection and atherosclerosis. JAMA 1989; 261:3561-3566.

26. Hruban RH, Wu TC, Beschorhner WE et al. Cytomegalovirus nucleic acids in allografted hearts (letter) Human Pathol 1990; 21:981-983.

27. Yamashiroya HM, Ghosh L, Yang R, Robertson AL. Herpesviridae in coronary arteries and aorta of young trauma victims. Am J Path 1988;1 30:71-79.

28. Hendrix MGR, Daemen M, Bruggeman CA. Cytomegalovirus nucleic acid distribution within the human vascular tree. Am J Path 1991; 138:563-567.

29. Pober JS. Cytokine-mediated activation of vascular endothelium, physiology and pathology. Am J Path 1988; 133:426-433.

30. Pober JS, Cotran RS. The role of endothelial cells in inflammation: Transplantation 1990; 50:537-544.

31. Pasternack MS, Medearis DN, Rubin RH. Cell-mediated immunity in experimental cytomegalovirus infections: A perspective. Rev Inf Dis 1990; 12:S720-S726.

32. Hruban R, Beschorner W, Baumgartner W et al. Accelerated arteriosclerosis in heart transplant recipients is associated with T-lymphocyte mediated endothelialitis. Am J Path 1990; 137:871-882.

33. Herskowitz A, Soule LM, Ueda K et al. Ateriolar vasculitis on endomyocardial biopsy: A histologic predictor of poor outcome in cyclosporin treated heart transplant recipients. Heart Transplant 1987; 6:127-136.

34. Palmer D, Tsai C, Roodman ST et al. Heart graft arteriosclerosis. Transplanation 1985; 39:385-388.

35. Salomon RN, Hughes CCW, Schoen FJ et al. Human coronary transplantation-associated arteriosclerosis. Am J Path 1991; 138:791-798.

36. Oguma S, Banner B, Zerbe TR et al. Participation of dendritic cells in vascular lesions of chronic rejection of human allografts. Lancet 1988: 933-936.

37. Kaufman C, Zeevi A, Kormos R et al. Propagation of infiltrating lymphocytes in heart and graft coronary disease in cardiac transplant recipients. Human Immunol 1990; 28:228-236.

38. Hess ML, Hastillo A, Mohanakumar T et al. Accelerated atherosclerosis in cardiac transplantation: Role of cytotoxic B-cell antibodies and hyperlipidemia. Circulation 1983; 68:II94-II101.

39. Reemtsra K. Vascular immunoobliterative disease: A common cause of graft failure. Transplant Proc 1989; 21:3706.

40. Alonso D, Starek P, Minick CR. Studies on the pathogenesis of atheroarteriosclerosis induced in rabbit cardiac allografts by the synergy of graft rejection and hypercholesterolemia. Am J Path

1977; 87:415-442.

41. Laden AMK. The effects of treatment on the arterial lesions of rat and rabbit cardiac allografts. Transplantation 1972; 13:281-290.

42. Hansson GK, Holm J, Jonasson L. Detection of activated T-lymphocytes in the human atherosclerotic plaque. Am J Path 1989; 135:169-175.

43. Hansson GK, Holm J, Kral JG. Accumulation of IgG and complement factor C3 in human arterial endothelium and atherosclerotic lesions. Acta Path Microbiol Immunol Scand 1984; 92:429-435.

44. Lopes-Virella MF, Virella G. Immunological and microbiological factors in the pathogenesis of atherosclerosis. Clin Immunol and Immunopath 1985; 37:377-386.

45. Yousem SA, Dauber J, Griffith B. Bronchial cartilage alteration in lung transplantation. Chest 1990; 98:1121-1124.

46. Yousem SA, Paradis I, Dauber J et al. Pulmonary arteriosclerosis in long term human heart-lung transplant recipients. Transplantation 1989; 47:564-569.

47. Griffith BP, Hardesty RL, Trento A. Heart-lung transplantation: Lessons learned and future hopes: Ann Thorac Surg 1987; 43:6.

48. Clelland CA, Higenbottom TW, Otulana BA et al. Histological grading of acute lung rejection on transbronchial biopsy helps predict long-term outcome of heart-lung transplants. Transplant Proc 1990; 22:1480.

49. Zeevi A, Keenan R, Duqeusnoy RJ. Lung transplantation: Bronchoalveolar lavage diagnosis of lung rejection. Critical Care Report 1991; 2:228-233.

50. Fend F, Prior C, Margreiter R, Mikuz G. Cytomegalovirus pneumonitis in heart-lung transplant recipients: Histopathology and clinical pathologic considerations. Human Pathol 1990; 21:918-926.

51. Hruban RH, Hutchins GM. Parallels between transplant related bronchiolitis obliterans and accelerated atherosclerosis. Cornotes 1991; 6:3-4.

52. Modry DL, Oyer PE, Jamieson SW et al. Cyclosporin in heart and heart-lung transplantation. Canad J Surg 1985; 28:274-282.

53. Uretsky BF, Kormos RL, Zerbe TR et al. The value of cornary arteriography in predicting cardiac events after heart transplantation. Abstract International Society of Heart Transplantation 1990

54. Glanville AR, Baldwin JC, Burke CM, Theodore J, Robin ED. Obliterative bronchiolitis post heart-lung transplantation: Apparent arrest by augmented immunosuppression. Ann Intern Med 1987; 107:300.

55. Ferns G, Reidy M, Ross R. Vascular effects of cyclosporine A in vivo and in vitro. Am J Path 1990; 137:403-413.

56. Cramer DV, Chapman FA, Wu G et al. Cardiac transplantation in the rat I. The effect of histocompatibility differences on graft arteriosclerosis. Transplantation 1989; 47:414.

57. Prop J, Tazelaar HD, Billingham ME. Rejection of combined heart-lung transplants in rats. Am J Path 1987; 127:97-105.

58. Ross R. The pathogenesis of atherosclerosis-an update NEJM 1986; 314:448-500.

59. Duquesnoy R, Trager JDK, Zeevi A. Propagation and characterization of lymphocytes from transplant biopsies. Crit Rev Immunol 1991; 10:455-80.

60. Taylor PM, Rose ML, Yacoub MH. Expression of mhc antigens in normal human lungs and transplanted lungs with bronchiolitis obliterans. Transplantation 1989; 48:506-510.

61. Lindner V, Lappi DA, Baird A, Majack RA, Reidy MA. Role of basic fibroblast growth factor in vascular lesion formation. Circ Res 1991; 68:106-113.

62. Xu CB, Falke P, Stavenow L. Interactions between cultured bovine arterial smooth muscle cells and endothelial cells: Studies on the release of growth inhibiting and growth stimulating factors. Artery 1990; 17:297-310.

63. Bell L, Madri JA. Influence of the angiotensin system on endothelial and smooth muscle cell migration. Am J Path 1990; 137:7-12.

64. Foegh ML. Chronic rejection-graft atherosclerosis. Transplant Proceed 1990; 22:119-122.

65. Martinet Y, Rom WN, Grotendorst GR et al. Exaggerated spontaneous release of platelet-derived growth factor by alveolar macrophages from patients with idiopathic pulmonary fibrosis. NEJM 1987; 317:202-209.

66. Palmiter R, Brinster R. Transgenic mice. Cell 1985; 41:343-345.

67. Jaenisch R. Transgenic animals. Science 1988; 240:1468-1474.

68. Nabel E, Plautz G, Boyce M, Stanley J, Nabel G. Recombinant gene expression in vivo within endothelial cells of the arterial wall. Science 1989; 244:1342-1344.

69. Wilson J, Birinyi L, Salomon R et al. Implantation of vascular grafts lined with genetically modified endothelial cells. Science 1989; 244:1344-1346.

70. Zwiebel J, Freeman S, Kantoff P. High-level recombinant gene expression in rabbit endothelial cells transduced by retroviral vectors. Science 1989; 243:220-222.

71. Rosenfeld M, Siegfried W, Yoshimura K et al. Adenovirus-mediated transfer of a recombinant alpha 1 antitrypsin gene to the lung epithelium in vivo. Science 1991; 252:431-434.

72. Rosenberg S, Aebersold P, Cornetta K et al. NEJM 1990; 323:570-578.

73. Anonymous. Doctors creating new pig breed to donate hearts to humans. Pittsburgh Press 1991.

74. Capecchi M. Altering the genome by homologous recombination. Science 1989; 244:1288-1292.

CHAPTER 8

NONINVASIVE DIAGNOSIS OF CARDIAC REJECTION

Maria-Teresa Olivari

The occurrence of acute graft rejection may soon become a reminiscence of the past due to the availability of new, better targeted immunosuppressive drugs and the development of techniques to induce immunotolerance in the human host. At the present time, however, acute graft rejection remains a major cause for morbidity and mortality in cardiac transplant recipients.

Since rejection in cyclosporine-treated patients has an indolent course without overt clinical signs of graft dysfunction until severe myocardial damage ensues, endomyocardial biopsy has become, during the last 10 years, the "gold standard" method for the early diagnosis of rejection. Several methods have been investigated in the search for noninvasive tests to diagnose rejection in cardiac transplant recipients. So far, none has been shown to be equal to endomyocardial biopsy for sensitivity and specificity. Nevertheless, major advances over the past few years in the field of nuclear radiology, nuclear magnetic resonance imaging and spectroscopy, and monoclonal antibody manufacturing attest to the possibility in the near future to routinely diagnose cardiac rejection with noninvasive techniques. Endomyocardial biopsy will be then used only to confirm histologically such a diagnosis.

During an episode of acute rejection the following processes take place:

1. Infiltration of the myocardium by T lymphocytes.
2. Disruption of sarcolemmal membrane and consequent exposure of intracellular macromolecules, e.g., myosin.
3. Vasculitis with resulting exudation, interstitial edema and decrease in myocardial blood flow and flow reserve.
4. Expression of class I and class II HLA antigens by myocardial and endothelial cells.
5. Changes in intracellular metabolism and pH.

The order in which the above processes take place is unknown. However, from animal studies, it appears that expression of HLA antigens precedes and is responsible for cellular and vascular damage and it is conceivable that changes in intracellular metabolism and in membrane integrity precede myocytolysis. The myocardial changes which occur during rejection can be assessed noninvasively by several techniques which I shall discuss. These techniques hopefully will soon allow us to accurately diagnose rejection noninvasively and furthermore, to assess in vivo its different stages thus increasing our understanding of this process.

In the normal, non-transplanted heart, myocytes and interstitial structures (vessels and dendritic cells) express no or very little HLA class I and class II antigens. A massive increase in class I antigen expression on myocardial cells and class II antigens on endothelial cells has been shown in the human transplanted heart to occur at time of rejection, to precede the appearance of lymphocytic infiltrates and myocytolysis by several days and to disappear after treatment. Persistent rejection has been characterized by continual myocardial expression of class I and II antigens. The antigens are donor-specific and in animals are not expressed when the myocardial damage is secondary to causes other than rejection. Monoclonal antibodies against human class I and class II antigens are now available. In the future, if appropriately radiolabeled, they can be used to obtain in vivo scintigraphic images of the heart for the diagnosis of rejection through the detection of expressed donor-specific antigens.

Myocardial cell damage or death results in loss of the cellular membrane integrity and inward diffusion of macromolecules. Antimyosin antibodies have been shown to bind to cardiac myosin when sarcolemmal membranes are disrupted as in myocardial infarction and myocarditis. Thus, areas of focal or diffuse myocyte damage can be scintigraphically identified in vivo by using Indium radiolabeled Fab fragments of monoclonal antimyosin antibodies. Since scattered necrosis of myocardial cells occurs even in mild rejection, antimyosin antibody scintigraphy has been recently used for the diagnosis of acute rejection in cardiac recipients with promising results. Quantitative evaluation of antimyosin uptake by determining the heart to lung uptake ratio appears to improve the specificity of the test and it has been useful particularly in the diagnosis of processes such as rejection and myocarditis which are usually characterized by diffuse, but low grade, myocyte damage. Studies in animals have suggested that myocyte damage is manifested by a defect in cellular membrane before morphological changes

occur. Therefore, scintigraphy with antimyosin antibodies should detect rejection in its earliest phases and quantification by the heart to lung ratio should allow grading of the severity of the process. Several technical problems are, however, limiting the current applicability of this technique.

1. Since the tracer clears slowly from the blood pool, the specificity of the test and the quality of images are markedly increased when scintigraphy is obtained 48 hours after antimyosin antibody administration. However, 48 hours represents an unacceptable delay in clinical practice.

2. The long half-life and high energy of Indium-111 limit the number of studies which can be performed in one individual. Use of different radionuclides with shorter half-lives will reduce the risk of serial studies.

Three additional problems have been suggested to exist specifically in transplanted animals.

1. Intravenous corticosteroids might decrease the uptake of antimyosin antibodies producing false negative results early after surgery and following treatment for acute rejection.

2. Cyclosporine might increase the permeability of the cellular membrane, thus producing false positive results.

3. Administration of therapeutic murine monoclonal antibodies such as OKT3 may induce human antimurine antibody formation which could potentially bind to the Indium-III labeled antimyosin antibodies rendering the test ineffective.

In the clinical studies performed to date, the use of these immunosuppressive agents appear not to have interfered with antimyosin imaging. However, further studies are necessary to assess whether or not this problem exists in human recipients and its magnitude.

During acute rejection, the coronary microcirculation is involved as documented by the presence of histopathologic changes such as swelling of endothelial cells, intimal proliferation, thrombosis, vascular necrosis, microinfarcts and interstitial edema. Coronary flow and coronary flow reserve, which in the absence of rejection are normal, decrease markedly during acute rejection. This reduction could be the result of (1) compression of microvessels by interstitial edema, (2) structural alterations of the vessels, (3) unresponsiveness of the vascular wall to vasodilator stimuli due to injury to the endothelial cells, or (4) decreased production of EDRF by injured endothelial cells. Whatever the cause(s), coronary flow and flow reserve normalize with treatment and resolution of rejection. Myocardial perfusion studies should be able to detect these alterations in coronary flow. In animal studies, a significant decrease in myocardial thallium uptake has been shown during rejection. Limited studies in human recipients have given contrasting results. Since coronary flow reserve is markedly impaired during rejection even when resting flow is preserved, the sensitivity of thallium imaging in detecting changes in myocardial perfusion during graft rejection should be enhanced by the administration of adenosine. So far, thallium-adenosine scintigraphy has not yet been investigated for the diagnosis of acute graft rejection. If proven to be specific and sensitive, it offers the advantages of safety, repeatability and quick results. The presence of graft atherosclerosis and/or left ventricular hypertrophy, both common in cardiac recipients, might, however, limit its accuracy to the early post-transplant period.

Nuclear magnetic resonance imaging and spectroscopy hold the greatest promise as noninvasive tests for the diagnosis of cardiac rejection since changes in myocardial water content, intracellular phosphorus metabolism and pH take place during rejection. These changes can be detected and monitored through these two techniques and their time course and extent, which are currently unknown in humans, can be monitored. In animal models of rejection, such changes occur prior to irreversible myocyte damage and prior to the appearance of histological changes. Magnetic resonance, therefore, might be of the greatest value for the early diagnosis of rejection. The considerable technological progress made during the last decade in the field of magnetic resonance attests to the imminent possibility to utilize in vivo spectroscopy associated with imaging for clinical purposes. In fact, the recent development of depth resolved surface coil spectroscopy (DRESS) and image-selected in vivo spectroscopy (ISIS) allow acquisition of in vi-

vo phosphorus spectra from volumes of tissue from a specific area of interest. When applied to the heart, the preselection of a volume of interest allows reduction of contamination from skeletal muscles and estimation of the relative volume occupied by the myocardium and the intracavitary blood.

The use of magnetic resonance imaging has been extensively investigated in several animal models of heterotopic cardiac transplant. Proton relaxation times (T_1 and T_2) increase significantly in the transplanted rejecting hearts while no changes in these two parameters are seen in the native hearts or in the transplanted hearts of immunosuppressed, nonrejecting animals. The increase in T_1 and T_2 parallels the increase in water content in the rejecting grafts and closely correlates with the severity of rejection by histology. Similar results have been obtained in few human studies when serial measurements were obtained. When an increase in proton relaxation times, T_1 and T_2, to more than two standard deviations above the normal values was considered diagnostic for rejection, the sensitivity and specificity of MRI have been found to be in excess of 90% and equal to endomyocardial biopsy. However, this technique has been shown to be inaccurate in recently transplanted patients (<1 month) since abnormal relaxation times after surgery can occur in the absence of rejection due to myocardial edema secondary to preservation injury. If in the future, NMR imaging were to be routinely combined with NMR spectroscopy, it should be possible to accurately diagnose rejection even shortly after surgery since it appears from preliminary studies in animal models that the changes in intracellular pH and metabolism which occur during rejection are qualitatively and quantitatively different from those due to ischemia.

^{31}P magnetic resonance spectroscopy, which now is not routinely available on commercial imagers, will surely be in the future. In animal studies, a significant decrease in phosphocreatinine (Pcr) and adenosine triphosphate (ATP) and increase in inorganic phosphate (Pi) have been observed in the early phases of rejection prior to the detection of histological changes. Pcr/ATP and Pcr/Pi ratios have been shown in animals to clearly separate rejecting from nonrejecting grafts. Moreover, in contrast to ischemia, which invariably produces a drop in pH, rejection does not produce a decrease in intracellular pH. This finding, if confirmed in humans, would allow investigation to differentiate metabolic changes early after transplant due to poor graft preservation from changes due to rejection. It might also be quite useful later after transplant should graft atherosclerosis develop.

SUMMARY

Although the incidence of acute graft rejection will decrease in the future and eventually rejection will be completely eliminated due to better immunosuppressive regimens, this goal will probably be achieved only a few decades from now. Meanwhile, new noninvasive methods to diagnose cardiac rejection are needed and will be investigated. Nuclear magnetic resonance imaging and spectroscopy and antibody scintigraphy, by assessing specific changes occurring in myocardial metabolism and structure early during rejection, hold the greatest promise in this field. If the current preliminary results are confirmed, with the constant technical progresses seen in imaging techniques, they will probably replace myocardial biopsy in the next decade and become the new "gold standard" procedures for the diagnosis of acute cardiac rejection in the near future.

CHAPTER 9

THE NONINVASIVE DETECTION OF LUNG REJECTION

John P. Scott

John Wallwork

The detection of lung rejection in man, largely parallels our understanding of the underlying immune processes involved. Ideally such techniques should be highly specific, though sensitive and should have high positive and low negative predicitivity so as to detect the developing rejection process so early as to pre-date tissue damage.

The management of acute lung rejection is based on the assumption that this is a discrete process in man. This a clinical concept, reflecting clinically detectable dysfunction and facilitates changes in maintenance immunosuppression and in directing the use of enhanced immunosuppression with intravenous steroids or antilymphocyte preparations. There is little to justify this concept from an immunological viewpoint. The tissue is always foreign to the host immune system and this concept of continous—if low grade—graft injury may have important implications for the development of long-term consequences of lung transplantation, such as obliterative bronchiolitis. However, it has been our practice to adhere to the clinically based definition of acute lung rejection and we shall do so in this text.

The historical role of histology in the confirmation of acute lung rejection was based largely on the pioneer work of Veith and coworkers.[1] More recently this has been extensively reclassified by Yousem and others.[2]

Whilst perivascular changes during clinical rejection have been helpful in confirming the diagnosis of lung rejection, such changes can be present without any clinical or physiological evidence of lung rejection.[3] They may however have significance in the evaluation of risk of developing obliterative bronchiolitis.[4,5]

The use of the transbronchial biopsy (TBB) technique in the diagnosis of acute rejection has been shown as feasible and effective in both adults[6] and in children as young as three years of age.[7] However, this technique does carry risks in patients who have severely impaired lung function as might occur during acute rejection or infection.[7] Although in our experience the risk of death has been approximately 0.1%, morbidity with bleeding and pneumothoracies is higher and it is clear that comparable noninvasive techniques should be sought.

CLINICAL INDICATIONS OF LUNG REJECTION

Acute lung rejection is characterized by dyspnea, tachypnea, fever and by occasional basal crepitations.[3,6,7] As such it is indistinguishable from viral, protozoan or fungal infection.

ROLE OF RADIOLOGY

Whilst the chest x-ray (CxR) is particularly valuable in the first three weeks after surgery during which time 70% of CxRs demonstrated rejection (as high as 94% in the first 10 days), the value of CxR in the long-term detection of rejection is poor, with at most 30% of biopsy confirmed rejection episodes beyond three months having radiological changes evident.[8] These figures in adults are little better in children.[7] The role of high resolution CT scan is uncertain, although it has potential for demonstrating the interstitial and/or alveolar infiltrates of more severe rejection.[9] As such it should prove superior to routine CxR, although more costly. However, in our experience neither method can reliably separate acute lung rejection from pulmonary infection. Nuclear scanning has to-date proved unhelpful, although Technicium scanning has demonstrated increased permeability in pneumocystis infection, but even in this condition, such a finding is nonspecific.[10]

PULMONARY PHYSIOLOGY

The role of forced expiratory volume in one second (FEV_1) in documenting the development of acute lung rejection has been extensively reported. If used to support the clinical evaluation of acute lung rejection this is relatively sensitive, specific (68%)[11] and permits home monitoring.[12] However, if compared with the pathology changes found in clinical rejection episodes the relationship is

weaker.[3] Again, a decline in FEV_1 does not exclude infection as a cause, although with sputum and blood culture, CxR and diffusing capacity and with appropriate antiprotozoan and antiviral prophylaxis, clinical evaluation may be possible. Two difficulties with this approach have been the failure of FEV_1 to fall with acute lung rejection in the first few months after transplantation, when instead a slowing of the usual rate of rise may be seen. Second, a decline in FEV_1 beyond six months may reflect irreversible loss of lung function with the onset of obliterative bronchiolitis.[4,5] Accordingly, FEV_1 is neither sensitive nor specific enough to provide a basis for the long-term management of lung transplant recipients, although it will remain a valuable adjuvant. Alternative approaches with specific airways resistance (SG_{AW}) or with forced expiratory flow between 25% and 75% of forced vital capacity (FEF_{25-75}) have been proposed, but neither is as robust a measurement as FEV_1, nor have either added significant specificity to such tests.[13]

SEROLOGICAL MARKERS OF LUNG REJECTION

BIOCHEMICAL MARKERS

A number of markers of the immune response have been proposed for the detection of acute rejection, including interleukin-2, interleukin-2 receptor, intercellular adhesion molecule-1, endothelial cell adhesion molecule-1, tumor necrosis factor and granulocyte membrane protein-140 (GMP-140).[14-19] Not all of these markers have yet been assessed for acute lung rejection, but all would seem capable of being so applied. All of these techniques represent an effort to amplify our detection of increased immune response, but not necessarily one of rejection, nor directed specifically against the lung rather than say infectious organisms, nor specific to the clinical syndrome. As a result specificity has been less than that found with TBB. As regards markers for rejection in other transplanted organs which merit application to the transplanted lung, there are a number of possibilities including prolactin,[20] noted to be helpful in cardiac rejection, urinary polyamines,[21] atrial naturetic factor (ANF)[22] noted to be elevated during rejection of heart-lung allografts in rats, neopterin[23] in heart transplant recipients, beta-2 microglobulin and serum amyloid A protein[24] in the kidney. Less likely to be helpful are acute phase reactant proteins such as alpha-1 macroglobulin, C-reactive protein, C3 and C4 components of complement and alpha-1 antitrypsin; with multivariate analysis unable to improve the specificity of such markers.[25]

ACTIVATED LYMPHOCYTES

Again, encouraging results have been seen for selected populations with this technique, but specificity is at best uncertain and the technique has to date been largely confined to one group.[26,27] Of particular interest with this technique has been the propagation and characterization of lymphocytes from transplant biopsies.[28] Our early experience with this technique has suggested that specificity is not high and that activation will occur with infection.

LAVAGE MARKERS OF LUNG REJECTION

The use of T cell subsets, activated lymphocytes and biochemical markers in lavage, has the advantage of organ specificity, the disadvantages of viability of sampling (technique, equipment, lung segment(s) used), variable dilution of sample and sample contamination as a result of induced bleeding. These disadvantages are usually apparent in the resulting low positive predictivity.[29]

IMPLICATIONS OF BLOCKING IL-2 OR IL-2R

Efforts both to block IL-2 with monoclonal antibody[30] and then to block IL-2R[31,32] have been well reported in the literature from two groups. Neither group has found this technique significantly superior to standard antilymphocytic therapy although fewer side effects were observed. Such findings support the view that IL-2 and its receptor, whilst important in the immune process are not the pivotal factors as once thought, and represent part of a more generalized immunological response.

MARKERS OF TISSUE INJURY

Suprisingly few recent reports have dealt with new techniques for the noninvasive diagnosis of lung tissue injury. Since transplanted organs are the overwhelmingly likely site of tissue injury in the transplant recipient, these markers may not have to be entirely specific to lung tissue. It may be sufficient to reflect injury to tissue types which are found in the lungs. This approach would then include the basement membrane protein laminin,[33] recently shown to be of value in detecting organ injury liver transplantation and fibrous matrix polysaccharides such as hyaluronic acid.[34]

PROSPECTS FOR THE FUTURE

If further improvements in the noninvasive detection of rejection are to be made, then the development of early organ specific markers of injury, the ability to separate rejection from other immunological responses and better understanding of the final pathway of cell destruction in rejection are required. The application of techniques reported in other transplanted tissues is awaited. However whilst development of these markers has increased our understanding of the immunology of rejection, these markers have not yet provided the support for the clinical syndrome of acute lung rejection that has been available through the critical evaluation of transbronchial lung biopsies.

REFERENCES

1. Veith FJ, Sinha SBP, Blumcke S et al. Nature and evolution of lung allograft rejection with and without immuno-suppression. J Thorac Cardiovasc Surg 1972; 63:509-20.
2. Yousem SA, Berry GJ, Brunt EM et al. A working formulation for the standardization of nomenclature in the diagnosis of heart and lung rejection: Lung rejection group. J Heart Transpl 1990; 9:593-601.
3. Scott JP, Higenbottam TW, Clelland CA, Smyth RL, Solis E, Wallwork J. A prospective study of 204 bronchoscopies in 52 heart-lung and lung transplant recipients using TBB. J Heart Transpl 1991; 10:626-36.
4. Scott JP, Higenbottam TW, Hutter J et al. The natural history of obliterative bronchiolitis. Transpl Proc 1991; 21:2592-3.

5. Scott JP, Higenbottam TW, Sharples L, Clelland CA, Mullins P, Smyth RS, Stewart S, Wallwork J. Risk factors for obliterative bronchiolitis in heart-lung transplant recipients. Transplantation 1991; 51:813-7.

6. Higenbottam TW, Stewart S, Penketh A, Wallwork J. Transbronchial lung biopsy for the diagnosis of rejection in heart-lung transplant patients. Transplantation 1988; 46:532-9.

7. Scott JP, Higenbottam TW, Smyth RL et al. Experience with TBB in children after heart-lung transplantation. Pediatrics 1990; 86:698-702.

8. Millett B, Higenbottam TW, Flower CDR, Stewart S, Wallwork J. The radiographic appearances of infection and acute rejection of the lung following heart-lung transplantation. Am Rev Resp Dis 1989; 140:62-67.

9. Genereux GP. CT of acute and chronic distal airspace (alveolar) disease. Semin Roentgenol 1984; 29:211-21.

10. Jones DK, Higenbottam TW. Pneumocystis carinii pneumonia increases the clearance rate of inhaled 99mTc DTPA from lung to blood. Chest 1985; 88:631-7.

11. Otulana BA, Higenbottam TW, Scott JP, Clelland CA, Igboaka G, Wallwork J. Lung function associated with histologically diagnosed acute lung rejection and infection in heart-lung transplant patients. Am Rev Resp Dis 1990; 141:329-332.

12. Otulana BA, Higenbottam TW, Ferrari L, Scott JP, Wallwork J. The use of home spirometry in detecting acute lung rejection and infection following heart-lung transplantation. Chest 1990; 97:353-7.

13. Schlick W, Salem G, Keiler A et al. Pulmonary function tests following single lung homotransplantation in emphasematous dogs. Res Exp Med 1975; 166:283-94.

14. Faull RJ, Russ GR. Tubular expression of intercellular adhesion molecule-1 during renal allograft rejection. Transplantation 1989; 48:226-30.

15. Lawrence EC, Holland VA, Young JB, Winsor NT et al. Dynamic changes in soluble interleukin-2 receptor levels after lung or heart-lung transplantation. Amer Rev Respir Dis 1989; 140:789-96.

16. Steinhoff G, Behrend M, Pichlmayr R. Induction of ICAM-1 on hepatocyte membranes during liver allograft rejection and infection. Transpl Proc 1990; 22:2308-9.

17. Sedmak DD, Orosz CG. The role of vascular endothelial cells in transplantation. Arch Pathol Lab Med 1991; 115:260-5.

18. Chang SC, Hsu HK, Perng RP, Shiao GM, Lin CY. Significance of biochemical markers in acute detection of canine lung allograft rejection. Transplantation 1991; 51:579-84.

19. McKenna RM, Schroeder TJ. Immunological monitoring in cyclosporine-treated patients. Clin Biochem 1991; 24:75-80.

20. Carrier M, Russell DH, Wild JC, Emery RW, Copeland JG. Prolactin as a marker of rejection in human heart transplantation. J Heart Transplantation 1987; 6:290-2.

21. Carrier M, Russell DH, Davis TP, Emery RW, Copeland JG. Urinary polyamines as markers of cardiac allograft rejection. A clinical evaluation. J Thoracic Cardiovasc Surg 1988; 96:806-10.

22. Haug CE, Shapiro JI, Cosby RL, Chan L, Weil R. Atrial naturetic factor (ANF) levels are elevated in rats bearing rejecting heart-lung allografts. Biochem Biophys Res Commun 1987; 146:625-9.

23. Havel M, Laczkovics A, Teufelbauer H, Muller MM, Wolner E. Neopterin as a new marker to detect acute rejection after heart transplantation. J Heart Transplant 1989; 8:167-70.

24. Maury CP, Teppo AM. Comparative study of serum amyloid-related protein SAA, C-reactive protein and beta-2 microglobulin as markers of renal allograft rejection. Clin Nephrol 1984; 22:284-92.

25. Hoszel WG, Havel M, Laczkovics A, Muller MM. Diagnostic validity of multivariate combinations of biochemical analytes as markers for rejection and infection in the follow up of patients with heart transplants. J Clin Chem Clin Biochem 1988; 26:667-71.

26. Dal-Cal RH, Zeevi A, Rabinowich H, Herland DB, Yousem SA, Griffith BP. Donor specific cytotoxicity testing: An advance in detecting pulmonary allograft rejection. Ann Thorac Surg 1990; 49:754-8.

27. Rabinowich H, Zeevi A, Paradis IL et al. Proliferative responses of bronchoalveolar lavage lymphocytesa from heart-lung transplant patients. Transplantation 1990; 49:115-21.

28. Duquesnoy RJ, Trager JD, Zeevi A. Propogation and characterization of lymphocytes from transplant biopsies. Crit Rev Immunol 1991; 10:455-80.

29. Shennib H, Ngugen D, Guttman RD, Mulder DS. Phenotypic expression of bronchoalveolar lavage cells in lung rejection and infection. Ann Thorac Surg 1991; 51:630-5.

30. Soulillou JP, Peyronnet P, LeMauff B et al. Prevention of rejection of kidney transplants by monoclonal antibody against interleukin-2. Lancet 1987; i:1339-42.

31. Soulillou JP, Cantaravich D, LeMauff B et al. Randomized controlled trial of a monoclonal antibody against the interleukin-2 receptor (33B3.1) as compared with rabbit antilymphocyte globulin for prophylaxis against rejection of renal allografts. New Eng J Med 1990; 322:1175-82.

32. Otto G, Thies J, Manner M et al. Monoclonal antibody to interleukin 2 receptor in liver graft rejection. Lancet 1990; 335:15496-7.

33. Reynes M, Tricottet V, Gugenheim JC, Hartman DJ, Szekely AM, Bismuth H. Modifications of biliary and vascular basement membrane laminin in serial hepatic biopsies after hepatic transplantation in man. Transplant Proc 1987; 19:2478-9.

34. Bjermer L, Engstrom-Laurent A, Lungren R, Rosenhall L, Hallgren R. Hyaluronate and type III procollagen peptide concentrations in bronchoalveolar lavage fluid in idopathic pulmonary fibrosis. Thorax 1989; 44:126-31.

CHAPTER 10

ANTIBIOTIC PROPHYLAXIS AND MANAGEMENT OF INFECTIOUS COMPLICATIONS

Stephen Dummer

INTRODUCTION

Over the last decade there has been a marked increase in the number of heart transplant operations performed; and for a number of years the major limiting factor in further growth has been the size of the donor pool. Lung transplantation has also emerged as a new clinical entity and made surprising strides given the current shortage of donors. Since survival rates appear to be improving in both heart and lung transplantation it is likely that the total pool of surviving patients with these transplants will rise for years before reaching a steady state. As a result an increasing number of physicians will be called upon to evaluate and provide care to heart or lung transplant recipients.

Infectious complications have been a part of heart transplantation since its inception. In the last 10 or 15 years major strides have been made in understanding and managing transplant infections and it is likely that we will see similar progress in the next 10 to 15 years. This review will first explore the important accomplishments of transplant infectious disease work of the last 15 years and then speculate freely about the changes that will take place in the next 15 years.

INFECTIOUS MORTALITY: NOW AND THEN

The first comprehensive study of infections after heart transplantation was published from Stanford in 1971. It documented a 25% mortality from infection in 20 patients. All deaths occurred during the first post-transplant year. Over the next decade of pioneering work at Stanford, the long-term (five year) actuarial mortality from infections was 40% making it more common than all other causes of death. Following the introduction of cyclosporine, infectious mortality fell.

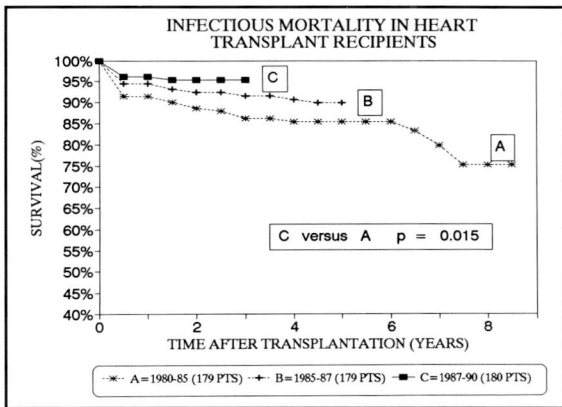

Fig. 1. Actuarial infectious mortality in three different sequential cohorts of heart transplant recipients at Pittsburgh. A = 179 patients (6/80-11/85); B = 179 patients (11/85-8/87); C = 180 patients (8/87-12/90) [Personal Communication: Robert Kormos].

Although much of this fall was attributed to superior characteristics of cyclosporine-based immunosuppression the actual reasons for the improvement in infectious mortality were probably complex and included a variety of medical improvements and innovations as well as ever-increasing diagnostic aggressiveness. Infectious mortality has continued to improve in the cyclosporine era. Figure 1 shows data on infectious mortality from 1980-1990 in the Pittsburgh heart transplant population. (personal communication: Dr. Robert Kormos) The population of 538 patients is divided into chronological thirds. From the earliest third (6/80-11/85) to the latest third (8/87-12/90) there is a significant fall in infectious mortality. The most recent infectious mortality was 4.5% at $3^1/_2$ years. If one excludes infectious deaths in patients in the mechanical heart program, who had a higher rate and severity of infections, the infectious mortality since 1985 is only slightly over 1% per year. Clearly the time may be approaching when one can aspire to the virtual elimination of infectious mortality after heart transplantation. Similar trends seem to be at play in lung transplantation although this group is still far away from achieving optimal control of infectious complications.

In the upcoming pages I shall review what I think are the main insights learned from the study of infections in transplant recipients, then describe a few of the more important recent technological achievements, and finally proceed to a prediction of the progress that is likely to be made in the next

Table 1. Important Concepts in Transplant Infectious Diseases

- Infections occur on a predictable time scale and vary with the type of transplant.

- Immunosuppression can be scientifically controlled

- The organ donor is an important source of infection

- Antibiotic prophylaxis is an important part of transplant management

10-15 years. The main conceptual achievements of the past are listed in Table 1. Although these points may seem obvious at present, they were not validated or even clearly thought out in the early years of transplantation.

ACHIEVEMENTS OF THE PAST

EPIDEMIOLOGY OF INFECTIONS

In 1981 Robert Rubin observed that the timing of infections after transplantation varied with the type of infecting pathogen. Thus symptomatic CMV infection was very frequent between 30 and 90 days after transplantation, whereas pneumocystis infection occurred most often between 60 and 180 days. Some other infections typically occurred late such as CMV retinitis, or cryptococcal infection. These paradigms derived from looking at transplant infection from an epidemiologic viewpoint. They form the basis of making differential diagnoses, structuring experimental studies and administering prophylaxis for infections. The actual epidemiology of infections varies somewhat with type of transplant and geographic region and hospital and probably with other factors such as the type or intensity of immunosuppression, so that each center also needs to look at its own experience with infections to derive the most benefit from this conceptualization.

IMMUNOSUPPRESSION

The observation that infection rates may vary with the type or intensity of immunosuppression has been often uttered but has required painstaking work to demonstrate. In a careful study in the 1970s, Mason found higher infection rates in patients who required ATG for rejection treatment. Other studies have shown an increased rate of fungal, protozoal or viral infections with OKT3. Increased steroid use has been shown to enhance fungal or viral infections. It is relatively recently that routine blood level measurements of an immunosuppressive drug have been done (cyclosporine). This practice of measuring serum levels of immunosuppressants will likely be a strong precedent for agents introduced in the future. A seemingly contrary, though perhaps allied trend has been the practice of using lower doses of multiple different immunosuppressive agents to achieve comparable immunosuppression with less toxicity. Other groups are trying to limit the use of corticosteroids primarily to the early postoperative period. The main achievement overall is the conceptual achievement that immunosuppression can be scientifically controlled by understanding mechanisms of action and pharmacokinetics and employing controlled doses of multiple focused agents.

DONOR TRANSMISSION

Transmission of CMV by renal allografts was demonstrated in the 1970s. Subsequently heart, liver and other allografts were also shown to transmit CMV infections. Two other important agents transmitted by heart allografts are *Toxoplasma gondii* and human

immunodeficiency virus. Hepatitis B virus and hepatitis C virus are also transmittable. Other agents transmitted by heart allografts appear to be of minor importance. Lung allografts may transmit subclinical bacterial and fungal infections that first become manifest in the recipient. Since the number of lung transplantations that have been performed is still relatively small, and since the lung is a target organ for a very broad range of pathogens it is likely that transmission of other important agents will be found. The knowledge that organs may transmit significant infections has made it possible to prospectively diagnose and more effectively treat or prevent these infections.

INCREASED USE OF PROPHYLAXIS

In the early days of thoracic transplantation prophylactic use of antibiotics was largely restricted to coverage for staphylococcal wound infections and topical anti-candidal therapy. From the mid-1980s onward there has been an increased interest in using prolonged postoperative prophylaxis for nonbacterial agents. Routine prophylaxis at many heart and lung transplant centers now includes routine sulfamethoxazole-trimethoprim prophylaxis against pneumocystis and also some form of antiviral prophylaxis against CMV, usually either oral acyclovir or intravenous immunoglobulin. Amazingly, there are few scientific studies documenting the efficacy of any prophylactic regimen in cardiac transplantation. Most of the regimens used have been validated in cancer patients or bone marrow and renal transplant populations. Standard perioperative antibacterial prophylaxis has been altered and extended in lung transplantation to include gram negative and anaerobic coverage because of the recognition that the donor lung is often subclinically infected. The use of prophylactic agents after transplantation needs to be better validated and refined but the greater use of prophylaxis appears to be permanent and is, I think a very positive trend.

IMPROVED DIAGNOSIS AND THERAPY

Although a host of new diagnostic techniques has been introduced over the last few years there have been relatively few that have had a significant impact on the infectious disease management of transplant recipients. The growth of scanning techniques such as CT scans has provided a means to image pathological anatomy throughout the body and is perhaps the most important advance. Other important developments have been the emergence of bronchoalveolar lavage as a diagnostic tool and the rapid antigen systems that allow detection of positive CMV cultures within one or two days. The discovery of Legionella organisms, the ongoing research into diagnostic techniques for Legionella and the identification of hospital water systems as a major source of endemic and epidemic infection have also been critical strides.

Since the mid-1970s there has been an outpouring of new antimicrobial agents. Most of the new agents have been antibacterial substances. The agents that have made the greatest impact in transplantation medicine, however, have been antiviral agents, particularly acyclovir and ganciclovir. Acyclovir has virtually eliminated herpes simplex virus infection as a significant problem and provided a nontoxic treatment for varicella zoster infections. Recent evidence also suggests that prophylaxis with high doses of acyclovir may reduce the morbidity from CMV infections after transplantation. The exact role of ganciclovir remains to be fully defined. It is enjoying wide use in solid organ transplantation. Although there is an emerging consensus that the drug is useful there is little consensus on how best to use it and further research will have to pinpoint its exact role. The only other agents that have aroused as much interest as the antiviral drugs are the newer oral antifungal agents such as fluconazole and itraconazole but it is still too early to say how important they will be.

DIRECTIONS FOR THE FUTURE

NEW OPERATIONS

The technique of heart transplantation is well-established. Technical problems are uncommon and not often associated with infection. Lung transplantation on the other hand is technically more demanding and in a state of flux at the present time. Technical problems in lung transplantation such as bleeding or anastomotic problems have been and continue to be associated with infectious complications. At the present time there appears to be a major trend towards the decreasing utilization of heart-lung procedures and widening the scope of single-lung transplantion. The infectious rates reported with this latter operation have been generally lower than with the heart-lung procedure. In the next 10 to 15 years we can expect further sophistication and technical ease in performing lung transplantation. Blood usage will be low for most single lung procedures and this should have a favorable impact on infection rates. At the same time late postoperative infections in the remaining native lung may be a problem especially if the lung is damaged by a process such as emphysema, that would normally be associated with a risk of infection. Mechanical heart technology should expand dramatically over the next 10 to 15 years. I think it is conceivable that $1/3$ to $1/2$ of all patients receiving heart transplants will wait with a mechanical heart in place. Many of these patients will have totally implantable devices and wait at home for transplantation. Although infections of these devices will still be a problem, intensive antibiotic prophylaxis, and improvements in materials technology and surgical care should reduce the frequency of these complications to a few percent or less. By the time 10 to 15 years have elapsed, the potency and selectivity of immunosuppression will have improved to the point where serious clinical trials of xenografting will be conducted. This experiment in xenografting will raise important and difficult infectious disease questions about the potential for the transmission of veterinary pathogens to man. These questions may be difficult to answer until the clinical experiments in man actually take place.

NEW TECHNOLOGY

Much of the future progress in transplant infectious diseases will emerge from the enormous capabilities of the molecular biology laboratory. The use of nucleic acid hybridization techniques such as the polymerase chain reaction (PCR) and monoclonal antibodies should provide the means to diagnose infections that have heretofore been difficult to study such as progressive multifocal encephalopathy. At the same time these techniques will also be applied quantitatively to the understanding of common transplant afflictions such as CMV infection. It will be particularly useful to have laboratory tools to rapidly assess viral load in such a way that one will be able to correlate levels of virus in organs or blood stream with clinical disease. These tools will also be extremely useful to assess response to antiviral therapy. In a like manner molecular techniques will be used to elucidate the still unclear association between Epstein-Barr virus infection and post-transplant lymphoproliferative disease and better means found to follow patients for Epstein-Barr virus infection than the currently used serologic assays. Probes will also be found and used for other difficult-to-diagnose entities such as invasive fungal infection due to aspergillus, candida and cryptococcus. Molecular probes and monoclonal antibodies will also find their way into the diagnosis of routine bacterial disease both in the detection of pathogens that are difficult to isolate such as chlamydia and mycoplasma and in the detection of genes or messenger RNA for drug resistance. In all these endeavors the thorough clinical evaluation and validation of the technology may be a more difficult and time-consuming task than its laboratory evolution.

New Antimicrobial Agents

Despite recent advances in the development of antimicrobial agents there are still a number of transplant infections that lack adequate therapy and others in which less toxic therapy is needed. Agents active against Aspergillus and oral agents active against CMV would be especially useful. It is likely that such agents will be found. Although the molecular basis for the latency of herpes viruses is not currently understood, within ten to twenty years molecular biology may be able to pinpoint the events that cause CMV

or herpes simplex infection to activate from latency. With this knowledge it may be possible to manipulate the molecular mechanism and down-regulate or even turn off viral reactivation entirely. It is certain that the struggle against microbes will not stop with classic antibiotics but will include molecules able to target virally-encoded antigens on infected cells and deliver destructive or inhibitory molecules directly to the cellular site of infection. It is hoped that therapy will not only be developed against common agents but also against infections such as adenovirus that are uncommon but currently untreatable. The trend to increased use of antibiotic prophylaxis will continue and include new and improved agents against all classes of organisms. Molecular probes will be developed that will aid in the detection of patients at risk for pneumocystis so that prophylaxis will be targeted at the population at risk for disease. Other probes will be used to detect infection due to *Toxoplasma gondii* in heart biopsies or blood stream before it becomes clinically apparent. Such diagnostic systems will also make discontinuation of prophylaxis easier because recrudescent infection will be easier to monitor. Even standard prophylaxis for wound infection is not likely to remain static. I would anticipate that in addition to new intravenous agents there will be a re-emergence of interest in topical prophylaxis.

Donor-Derived Disease

It almost certain that further diseases transmitted by donor organs will be found. Panels of probes will be developed to search for such agents so that their transmission can either be avoided or treated by antimicrobial therapy. CMV infection will initially be managed with antibiotic prophylaxis or treatment but with time there will also be increasing enthusiasm for donor/recipient CMV matching to prevent infection in CMV seronegative recipients. Such a policy has in fact already been introduced by the Papworth Heart and Lung Transplant group in Cambridge, England. In order for this approach to be accepted in the United States, feasibility studies will have to be done on a regional or national basis. With time and collection of data the advantages of this approach will emerge and be widely accepted.

NEW IMMUNOSUPPRESSIVE AGENTS

Ultimately the frequency and severity of infectious complications of transplantation depend on the degree of selectivity of the immunosuppression used. Ideal immunosuppression should inhibit only the immune response against foreign determinants, but leave other immune responses untouched. The HLA system is extremely polymorphic and the immune response against it highly sensitive to minor changes, even of single amino acids. Nonetheless the ability to block specific immune responses or selectively delete clones of lymphocytes having a recognition or cytotoxic role at specific epitopes may well be within the grasp of molecular immunology. Antigen-specific immunosuppression should be a long term goal and might indeed obviate the need for special infectious disease input in the transplant setting.

GOALS FOR THE FUTURE

Although infections after heart transplantation will not be eliminated as a problem in the foreseeable future, death rates due to infection could be brought to 1% per year or less within the next decade or two. Similar results will be more difficult to achieve in lung transplant recipients in part because of the susceptibility of the transplanted lung to infection and in part because of the inevitable secondary infectious complications of severe bronchiolitis obliterans. Ultimately progress in lung transplantation will probably depend on better prophylactic regimens than we now possess and on the means to control the progression of bronchiolitis.

REFERENCES

1.　Balfour HH, Chace BA, Stapleton JT et al. A randomized, placebo-controlled trial of oral acyclovir for the prevention of cytomegalovirus disease in recipients of renal allografts. N Engl J Med 1989; 320:1381-1387.

2.　Dummer JS, Hardy A, Poorsattar A, Ho M. Early infections in kidney, heart, and liver transplant recipients on cyclosporine. Transplantation 1983; 36:259-267.

3.　Eisenstein BI. The polymerase chain reaction. N Engl J Med 1990; 322:178-82.

4.　Gleaves CA, Smith TF, Shuster EA, Pearson Gr. Comparison of standard tube and shell vial cell culture techniques for the detection of cytomegalovirus in clinical specimens. J Clin Microbiol 1985; 21:217-221.

5.　Fleischhauer K, Kernan NA, O'Reilly RJ, Dupont B, Yang SY. Bone marrow-allograft rejection by T lymphocytes recognizing a single amino acid difference in HLA-B44. N Engl J Med 1990; 1818-22.

6.　Gottesdiener KM. Transplanted infections: Donor-to-Host transmission with the allograft. Ann Intern Med 1989; 110:1001-1016.

7.　Griffith BP. Interim use of Jarvik-7 artificial heart. Ann Thorac Surg 1989; 74:158-66.

8.　Grossman RF, Frost A, Zamel N et al. Results of single-lung transplantation for bilateral pulmonary fibrosis. N Engl J Med 1990; 322:727-33.

9.　Hanto DW, Frizzera G, Gajl-Peczalska KJ, Simmons RL. Epstein-Barr Virus, immunodeficiency, and B cell lymphoproliferation. Transplantation 1985; 39:461-72.

10.　Hofflin JM, Potasman I, Baldwin JC, Oyer PE, Stinson EB, Remington JS. Infectious complications in heart transplant recipients receiving cyclosporine and corticosteroids. Ann Intern Med 1987; 106:209-216.

11.　Kahan BD. Individualization of cyclosporing therpay using pharmacokinetic and pharmacodynamic parameters. Transplantation 1985; 40:457-476.

12.　Deay S, Bissett J, Merigan TC. Ganciclovir treatment of cytomegalovirus infections in iatrogenically immunocompromised patients. J Infect Dis 1987; 156:1016-21.

13.　Mason JW, Stinson EB, Hunt SA, Schroeder JS, Rider AK. Infections after cardiac transplantation: Relation to rejection therapy. Ann Intrn Med 1976; 85:69-72.

14.　Muder RR, Yu VL, Woo AH. Mode of transmission of legionella pneumophila. Arch Intern Med 1986; 146:1607-11.

15.　Pennock JL, Oyer PE, Reitz BA et al. Cardiac transplantation in perspectiver the future. J Thorac Cardiovasc Surg 1982; 83:168-177.

16.　Renlund DG, O'Connell JB, Gilbert EM et al. Feasibility of discontinuation of corticosteroid maintenance therapy in heart transplantation. J Heart Transplant 1987; 6:71.

17.　Rubin RH, Wolfson JS, Cosimi AB, Tolkoff-Rubin NE. Infection in the renal transplant recipient. Am J Med 1981; 70:405-411.

18.　Snydman DR, Werner BG, Heinze-Lacey B et al. Use of cytomegalovirus immune globulin to prevent cytomegalovirus disease in renal-transplant recipients. N Engl J Med 1987; 317:1049-54.

19. Singh N, Dummer JS, Kusne S et al. Infections with cytomegalovirus and other herpesviruses in 121 liver transplant recipients: Transmission by dontated organ and the effect of OKT3 antibodies. J Infect Dis 1988; 158:124-131.

20. Shields AF, Hackman RC, Fife KH et al. Adenovirus infections in patients undergoing bone-marrow trasnplantation. N Engl J Med 1985; 312:529-533.

21. Stinson EB, Bieber CP, Griepp RB, Clark DA, Shumway NE, Remington JS. Infectious complications after cardiac tranpslantation in man. Ann Intern Med 1971; 74:22-36.

22. Stover DE, Zaman MB, Hajdu SI, Lange M, Gold J, Armstrong D. Bronchoalveolar lavage in the diagnosis of diffuse pulmonary infiltrates in the immunosuppressed host. Ann Intern Med 1984; 101:1-7.

23. Wreghitt TG, Hakim M, Gray JJ et al. Toxoplasmosis in heart and heart and lung transplant recipients. J Clin Pathol 1989; 42:194-199.

CHAPTER 11

VIROLOGIC DIAGNOSIS AND TREATMENT

Jeffrey D. Hosenpud

INTRODUCTION

Viral disease in the allograft recipient is currently responsible for a variety of both acute and chronic disease states and continues to result in significant morbidity and mortality.

In addition, viral disease appears to be responsible for the majority of post-transplant lymphoproliferative disease and is implicated as a contributing mechanism in the development of cardiac allograft vasculopathy, the most common cause of late morbidity and mortality. This chapter reviews what is currently understood and postulated about specific etiologic agents and the resulting diseases, current and potential future methodologies of viral diagnosis and finally approaches to antiviral therapy.

POST-TRANSPLANT VIRAL DISEASES—DOCUMENTED AND PRESUMED

The majority of important post-transplant viral diseases are the result of either transmission of the infectious agent with the allograft or reactivation of a latent viral infection secondary to immunosuppression. In either instance the manifestation of the disease is substantially impacted by the host's immune status. The viral disease can manifest as an acute illness, a chronic persistent viral infection or a chronic disease presumably mediated by viral transformation of host cells. (Table 1)

CYTOMEGALOVIRUS

Clearly the most important viral disease manifesting in the post-transplant period is cytomegalovirus (CMV). The incidence of cytomegalovirus infection in the normal population is extremely high and varies from 50 to 75% depending on the geographic area. The infection occurs in one of three ways. First and usually most severe is the primary infection which results from the transplantation of an organ from a CMV positive donor to a recipient without a prior exposure to CMV. Second is the

Table 1. Viral Agents and Post-Transplant Disease

Agent	Manifestations
Herpes Viruses	
Cytomegalovirus	•Acute–"Mono-like" Syndrome, Pneumonitis, Hepatitis, Gastro-enteritis, Chorioretinitis •Chronic–? Renal Dysfunction, ? Cardiac Allograft Vasculopathy
Epstein-Barr	•Acute– "Mono-like" Syndrome, Hepatitis •Chronic–Post Transplant Lymphoma, Lymphoproliferative Disease
Herpes Simplex	Localized Mucus Membranes, Potential for Dissemination
Varicella Zoster	Localized Skin, Potential for Dissemination
Herpes Virus 6	? True Pathogen
Retroviruses	
HIV-1	AIDS
HTLV1	Leukemia/Lymphoma
Hepatitis Viruses	
Hepatitis B	Acute and Chronic Hepatitis
Hepatitis C	Acute and Chronic Hepatitis
Papilloma Viruses	Verrucae

reactivation of latent virus in the recipient as the result of the immunosuppressed state. Finally, a recipient can be infected with a second strain of CMV from the donor despite having had prior exposure to CMV. The latter two mechanisms of disease are at times difficult to distinguish especially if both the donor and the recipient are CMV positive, and both tend to manifest as a less severe disease compared to the primary infection and frequently are asymptomatic.[1]

The most common manifestations of acute CMV disease include fever, chills and malaise. Tissue invasion can occur in several sites including the lung, manifesting as a bilateral interstitial pneumonitis, the liver, presenting as a usually mild hepatitic picture, and the gastrointestinal tract with ulceration and gastrointestinal bleeding. Other sites of tissue invasion include the retina, skin and skeletal muscle.[1,2,3] Rarely has CMV myocarditis been reported.[4] Tissue invasive CMV until very recently carried a mortality of as high as 80% in some series.[2] Following the acute illness, a small proportion of patients will not completely clear the infection and chronically shed CMV in the urine. The site of chronic infection is felt to be the kidney, as blood buffy coat cultures are rarely positive, and the infection may contribute to progressive renal dysfunction occasionally seen in these patients.[5] A most worrisome recent finding is the association between CMV disease and the chronic coronary vascular disease[6] in this review referred to as cardiac allograft vasculopathy (CAV). If this association is in fact valid, as CAV is restricted solely to the allograft, one must hypothesize some interaction between the virus and alloimmunity. One hypothesis is that the virus by infecting some component of the vascular wall results in an alteration in alloantigenicity and immunologic recruitment directed against the coronary artery producing a cascade of events resulting in the myointimal proliferative lesions identified with CAV. (Fig. 1) We have recently reported that endothelial cells are poorly permissive for at least the early events of CMV infection in vitro and hence may not be the target tissue for CMV.[7] In contrast, smooth muscle cells are extremely permissive for the early events of CMV infection in vitro. Furthermore, the density of major histocompatibility complex cell surface antigens is regulated on these smooth muscle cells as a result of this infection. Unfortunately, at least preliminary data suggests that smooth muscle cells do not elicit a lymphocyte proliferative response and therefore might not be capable of presenting

antigen. Based upon the above preliminary data, one would therefore have to speculate that some paracrine signal between the smooth muscle cell and the endothelial cell would result in an alteration in the endothelial cell alloantigenicity and ultimately, a smooth muscle cell proliferative response as a result of immunologic attack.

OTHER HERPES VIRUSES

Epstein-Barr Virus (EBV). Acute primary EBV infections are unusual following transplantation and when they occur present similarly to the acute presentations in non-immunosuppressed individuals. The major morbidity of EBV in the transplant population is a result of the ability of the virus to transform host cells. The vast majority of post-transplant lymphoproliferative disease[5] and lymphoma[5] are B cell derived, range from polyclonal lympho-

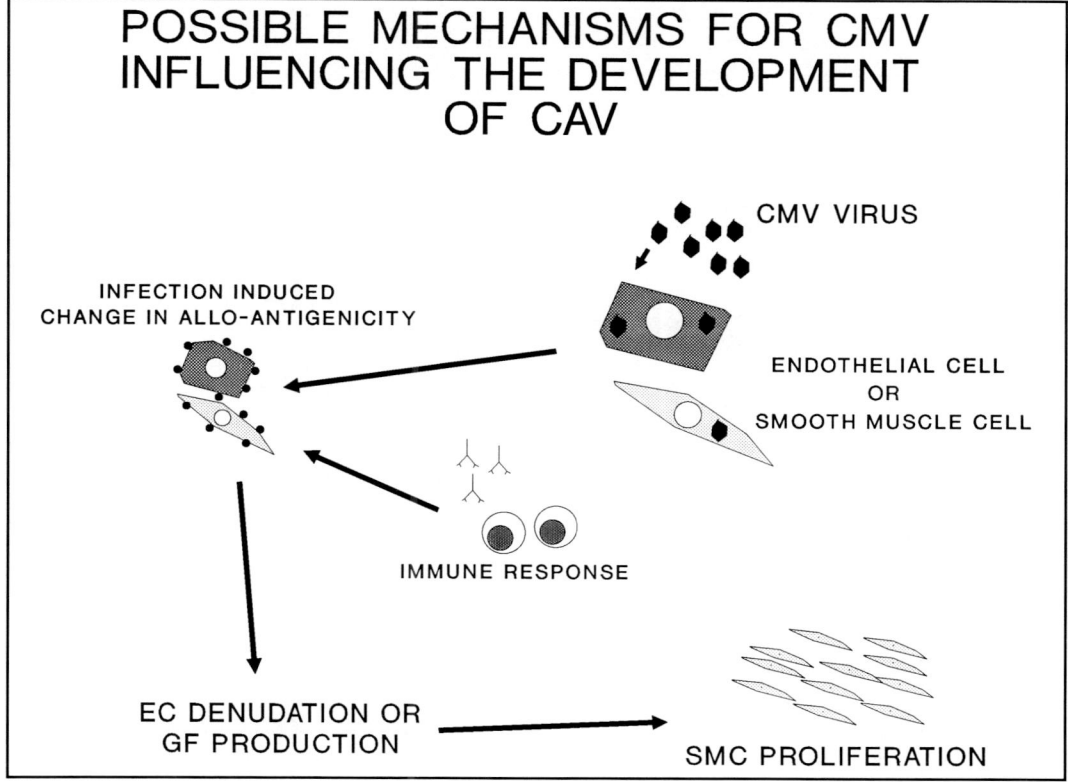

Fig. 1. A schema for a possible mechanism by which cytomegalovirus (CMV) influences the development of cardiac allograft vasculopathy CAV. The virus infects one of the cellular constituents of the vascular wall leading to a change in expression of cell surface antigen (MHC or other) leading to altered alloantigenicity. This elicits an increased immunologic response resulting in cell death or activation and smooth muscle cell growth factor production.

proliferation to true monoclonal lymphoma[5] and in some cases portions of the tumor have both polyclonal and monoclonal features. In most, the EBV DNA can be identified.[8] Tumors occurring within the first few months following transplantation are more likely to be polyclonal whereas tumors occurring later are more likely monoclonal.[9] Other unique features of the post-transplant lymphoproliferative disease and lymphomas include a high incidence of extranodal primary disease and their response, in many cases, to a reduction of immunosuppression.[10]

Herpes Simplex. Reactivation of both oral and genital Herpes simplex is common following transplantation and immunosuppression and most common during or shortly after intensification of immunosuppression for rejection. In the vast majority of cases, the virus remains localized although healing is usually slower than in the nonimmunosuppressed host. There is always the potential of dissemination and for this reason, most centers actively treat even localized lesions.

Varicella zoster. As with Herpes simplex, almost all cases are a reactivation of latent virus. The danger of dissemination is however greater than with H. simplex, and with dissemination (especially pneumonitis) the mortality is high. All cases therefore require high-dose acyclovir therapy.

Herpes Virus 6 (HS6). HS6 is responsible for the acute pediatric febrile illness roseola. It is manifest by a short febrile illness followed by a fine erythematous rash. No other sequela are known. HS6 is now receiving considerable interest in the post-transplant population however its role in producing disease is unclear. It has been suggested as an etiologic agent for a variety of syndromes including non-EBV lymphomas and hepatitis, although evidence for any association with disease is not available. Virtually 100% of the population has positive serology for HS6, however in only around 10% of the transplant population can the virus be isolated or part of the viral genome identified using extremely sensitive techniques (polymerase chain reaction). The overall incidence of reactivation is at this time unknown.

Human Immunodeficiency Virus (HIV-1). HIV mediated disease post-transplantation has been rarely reported and thus far the principle mechanisms have been the transmission of the virus with the transplanted organ or the transplantation of an unknown carrier.[11] The virulence of the disease may be exacerbated by immunosuppression and is especially severe in adults in contrast to children. Although screening of donors is now uniform, the window between infection and serologic positivity still allows for the potential of undetected infection. This would also be the case for screening potential recipients (routinely done in most transplant programs). It is anticipated that increasingly sensitive techniques to diagnose the virus in the donor at earlier stages will ultimately eliminate this problem. The difficulty with increasing the sensitivity of any technique is that one almost always sacrifices specificity, thus potentially impacting on an already scarce donor supply. One would hope and anticipate that with improving technologies especially in the molecular area, both sensitivity can be increased and specificity retained.

HEPATITIS VIRUSES

Hepatitis B. The outcome of renal allografting and more recently hepatic allografting in patients positive for hepatitis B surface antigen has been the subject of several reports.[12-14] Some have suggested that graft survival is not compromised in this population compared to patients without hepatitis B, although viral reactivation is common.[13] In contrast, primary infection post-transplant, presumably secondary to either blood or the donor organ has been associated with severe hepatic disease.[12] As with HIV, hepatitis B is routinely screened for by organ procurement agencies, but also as with HIV, a window between infection and positive serology is present.

Hepatitis C. Previously grouped in those cases referred to as non A, non B hepatitis, hepatitis C likely accounts for at least 50% of undiagnosed cases of hepatitis. The natural history of this disease is unclear given the very recent ability to diagnose the specific virus. Screening methods are quite sensitive but notoriously nonspecific (as low as 50% specificity) again leading to the potential wasting of organs.[15] It is not clear if those recipients receiving organs from donors with documented hepatitis C actually develop disease and at what rate. Early reports suggest that in those patients who become hepatitis C antibody positive the disease is usually mild both in the acute and chronic phases.[16]

CURRENT AND FUTURE METHODOLOGIES IN VIRAL DIAGNOSIS

SEROLOGY

The traditional method for the diagnosis of viral disease utilizes the host's humoral response to the infection. Antibodies to specific viral antigens can be detected by a variety of methodologies including complement fixation, immunofluorescence, ELISA, latex agglutination, indirect hemaglutination and radioimmunoassays.

Moreover, there are ELISA assays available to measure both IgG and IgM antibodies, allowing for the determination of whether or not a given infection was recent. The newer methodologies such as ELISA for CMV are easy to perform, at least as accurate as the complement fixation assays and the results are relatively quickly available.[17] Radioimmunoassys are extremely sensitive, but more cumbersome to perform. The difficulty with all serologic techniques are that they rely on the host's immune response and are therefore only positive well into the acute illness (days to weeks), and in the case of IgG levels remain positive for long periods of time. Nonetheless they are extremely important in such applications as matching donors and recipients for prior CMV infection, screening donors for prior or current viral infections (HIV, hepatitis) and evaluating and risk stratifying potential recipients. It would be anticipated that serologic techniques will continue to be improved both in sensitivity and specificity and in ease and rapidity of performance. The increase in sensitivity for a variety of illnesses such as HIV and the hepatitis viruses is important to donor evaluation so that the window between infection and serologic response can be shortened. The increase in specificity is absolutely essential to avoid the wasting of organs (as potentially could be the case for hepatitis C). Finally, as organ donation becomes

more and more complicated with multiple retrieval teams involved, the speed at which these assays can be performed and the body fluids/blood required will be extremely important to this process.

VIRAL ISOLATION

Actual viral isolation is the most definitive diagnostic evidence, of all assays available, for the etiology of an acute infection. Even this evidence is not, however, absolute, as virus, notably CMV, can be present as a colonization

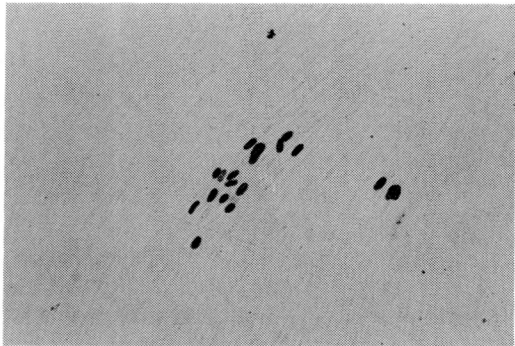

Fig. 2. Identification of CMV infection on a fibroblast monolayer using the peroxidase-labeled monoclonal antibody L-14 against the CMV immediate-early antigen. The infected fibroblasts demonstrate dark staining nuclei. [Courtesy of Sunwen Chou, M.D., Division of Infectious Diseases, Veteran's Affairs Hospital, Portland, Oregon]

along with another infectious agent. For CMV, until very recently, viral culture required the development of cytopathic changes in a fibroblast monolayer, an event which can take on the average 1 to 2 weeks. Less important previously, but with the current and future development of active antiviral agents, rapid diagnosis, within the first 24-48 hours becomes much more critical.

An extremely important advance in the diagnosis of CMV disease was the development of monoclonal antibodies to a 72-kDa CMV antigen which is expressed within the first 24 hours of infection.[17] Virus cultures from buffy coat, urine, broncho-alveolar lavage or other body fluid are set up on flat fibroblast monolayers on coverslips in shell vials.

After approximately 16 hours, the fibroblast monolayers are stained with the specific

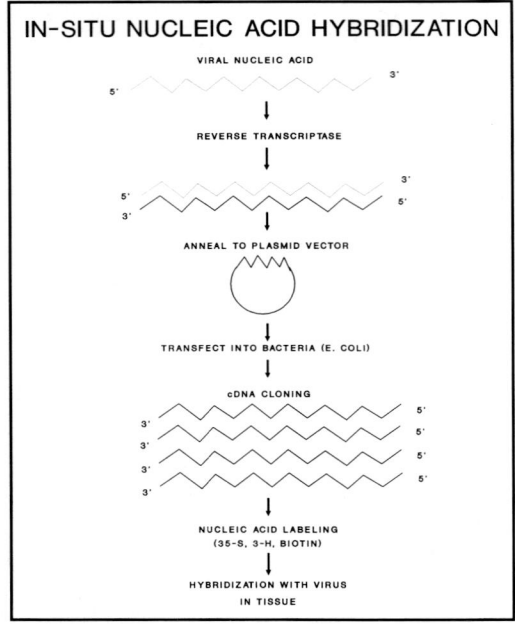

IN-SITU NUCLEIC ACID HYBRIDIZATION

VIRAL NUCLEIC ACID

REVERSE TRANSCRIPTASE

ANNEAL TO PLASMID VECTOR

TRANSFECT INTO BACTERIA (E. COLI)

cDNA CLONING

NUCLEIC ACID LABELING
(35-S, 3-H, BIOTIN)

HYBRIDIZATION WITH VIRUS
IN TISSUE

Fig. 3. In situ nucleic acid hybridization is demonstrated in this schematic. A complementary strand of DNA is synthesized to viral nucleic acid using a reverse transcriptase enzyme. This newly synthesized cDNA is then annealed to a plasmid vector and transfected into bacteria. The bacteria then replicate producing multiple copies of the cDNA which are then isolated, labeled and incubated with the target tissue. Any matching viral nucleic acid will then hybridize with the labeled cDNA, allowing identification.

monoclonal antibody using an immunoperoxidase procedure and the nuclei of the CMV infected cells stain with a dark reddish color. (Fig. 2) This technique is now available in most transplant centers. One would anticipate similar techniques becoming available as a whole host of viral agents become better characterized and monoclonal antibodies developed.

VIRAL IDENTIFICATION IN TISSUE

The identification of virus or viral effects in tissue had up until very recently been very limited. Under light microscopy, one can only rely upon characteristic cytopathologic changes (inclusion bodies with CMV). Electron microscopy is capable of identifying virus or viral particles, but has not been practical in clinical virologic diagnosis. Only with the development of newer molecular biologic techniques has both sensitive and specific viral identification in tissue become a reality. The ultimate clinical use of these techniques, however, is yet to be defined.

In Situ Nucleic Acid Hybridization. The principals of this technique are outlined in Figure 3. Briefly, with the knowledge of the viral genome, a complementary DNA chain (cDNA) to a portion of the genome can be synthesized and cloned using standard DNA cloning techniques. The cloned cDNA can then be labeled with any one of a number of tags to permit detection. The

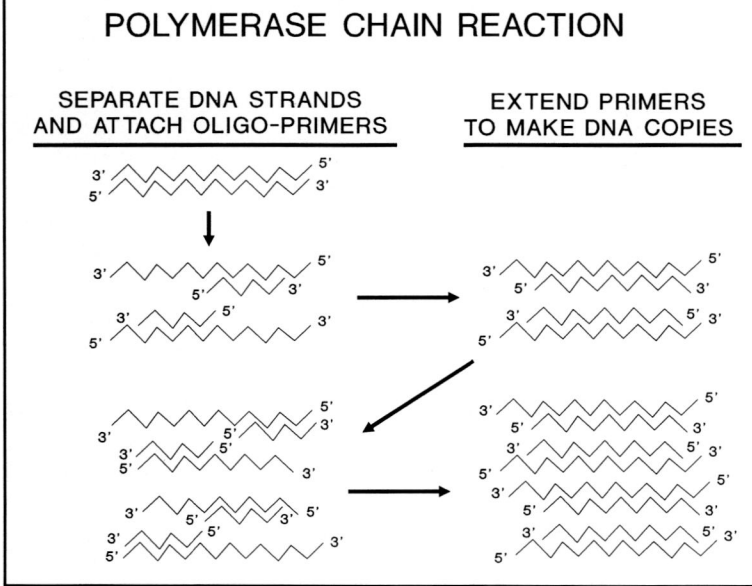

POLYMERASE CHAIN REACTION

SEPARATE DNA STRANDS AND ATTACH OLIGO-PRIMERS

EXTEND PRIMERS TO MAKE DNA COPIES

Fig. 4. The polymerase chain reaction (PCR) is now commonly utilized to amplify specific, in this case viral, DNA. By using amplification primers of between 15 and 25 oligonucleotides in length that are specific to the viral genome of interest, one can cycle through DNA dissociation, annealing and synthesizing temperatures and create DNA copies at an exponential rate (see text).

most sensitive methods utilize a radioactive label such as ^{35}S, and with this label may be able to detect as little as 10 viral genomic copies within a given cell. The radiolabeled cDNA is then incubated with the target tissue and binding to the complementary viral nucleic acid is detected using autoradiographic techniques. Probes to several viruses including CMV and coxsackie have been developed,[17,18] and many are commercially available.

DNA Amplification. An alternative to visually identifying viral genome in a tissue specimen, is the isolation and amplification of portions of the viral genome in vitro.[19] This is now relatively easily accomplished using the polymerase chain reaction (PCR). The technique is briefly outlined in Figure 4.

Amplification primers of between 15 and 25 nucleotides are synthesized to complement specific regions of the viral genome. It is important that the regions chosen are unique to the given virus of interest so that host DNA or other viruses do not cross react. A unique enzyme, the Taq polymerase, has made PCR technology possible on an automated scale. This enzyme isolated from the thermophillic bacteria *Thermus aquaticus* has the property of becoming active at approximately 70°C, able to withstand temperatures required for dissociating double stranded DNA (95°C) without denaturing and becoming inactive at DNA annealing temperatures of around 55°C. Tissue, blood or other body fluids are made into crude lysates, the appropriate oligonucleotide amplification primers and the Taq polymerase are added and the reaction mixture is then cycled through various temperatures using a programmable temperature block. At temperatures above 90°C the double stranded DNA is dissociated during cooling (to around 50°C), the primers anneal to the target DNA (or RNA) and at approximately 70°C the polymerase is active and synthesizes new complementary chains of DNA. This cycle can be repeated through multiple cycles with the original target DNA being amplified exponentially at each cycle. Theoretically, a single viral genome could be detected with this technology. Furthermore, the entire process including identification of the synthesized product will likely be automated in the near future.

Table 2. Methods of Viral Diagnosis

Serology
    Complement Fixation
    IgM Assays
    Neutralizing Antibodies
    Latex agglutination
    Immunofluorescence
    Radioimmunoassays

Viral Culture
    Traditional Methods
    Culture and Detection of Early Antigen

Viral Detection
    Antigen Detection (monoclonal Abs)
    Nucleic Acid Hybridization
    DNA Amplification

APPLICATIONS OF NEW TECHNOLOGIES

Table 2 summarizes the currently utilized diagnostic methodologies. It is clear that with the newer technologies, virus in a given clinical specimen will be able to be detected at extremely high sensitivities and specificities and with greater ease and rapidity. As most of these new technologies utilize the identification of all or portions of the viral genome, the limitations will relate to whether the identified viral sequences are complete and hence able to result in intact virions. These limitations should improve with technical refinements and better understanding of viral life cycles in various tissues.

These techniques will likely have direct impact on donor organ allocation, recipient risk profiling, diagnosis of acute infection and the early identification of virus associated with chronic morbidity. For instance, it is not clear why some CMV seropositive organ donors transmit CMV infection and others do not.[20] A marker for infective CMV virion in donor organs would provide this data allowing for the potential use of prophylactic therapy. The ability to absolutely rule out HIV and hepatitis because techniques are sensitive enough to detect one or two virions will allow for the IV drug user to become a potential organ donor. The early detection of EB virus may permit therapy to prevent post

Table 3. Current Antiviral Therapy

Active Immunization
>   Influenza
>   Rubeola
>   Rubella
>   Polio
>   Hepatitis B

Passive Immunization
>   Gamma Globulin
>   Hepatitis Hyperimmune Globulin
>   CMV Hyperimmune Globulin

Antivirals
>   Amantidine
>   Acyclovir
>   Ganciclovir

transplant lymphomas and lymphoproliferative disease, and the identification of viral-mediated vascular disease will again allow for potential early therapeutic intervention.

CURRENT AND FUTURE APPROACHES TO ANTIVIRAL THERAPY

Specific antiviral therapy continues to be quite limited with a few recent exceptions. (Table 3) Active immunization for influenza, hepatitis B and pediatric illnesses such as polio, rubella and rubeola are effective pretransplantation, but live-attenuated virus is contraindictated and the efficacy of killed virus vaccination is less clear in the immunosuppressed host. Furthermore, we have recently presented evidence that active influenza immunization may alter alloreactivity following cardiac transplantation.[21]

Passive immunization with immune globulin may be effective in hepatitis A and may blunt the severity of disease following cytomegalovirus infection.[22] Its use in the prophylactic setting is still under investigation. It is quite unlikely that significant advances will be made in the area of passive immunization.

Active antiviral agents include amantidine which has activity against some strains of influenza, acyclovir which is active against Herpes simplex, Varicella zoster and possibly Epstein-Barr virus and most recently ganciclovir which appears to be quite active against CMV. Acyclovir is well tolerated and is used extensively to pre-

vent dissemination of localized disease. It also appears to reduce the time of viral replication and speeds lesion healing. Finally, there has been some interest and positive experience using high dose acyclovir as part of the treatment for EBV associated lymphoma and lymphoproliferative disease, however this experience is quite limited to date.[23]

Invasive CMV, especially with lung involvement carried a mortality risk of as high as 80% prior to the availability of ganciclovir.[1] There are now several reports in the literature demonstrating a marked reduction in this mortality with the use of ganciclovir.[24,25] It is available only in the intravenous form, but is extremely well tolerated. Studies using an oral form of ganciclovir are currently in progress. Recent studies using prophylactic ganciclovir in allograft recipients at high risk for primary CMV appear to also demonstrate a beneficial effect both in reducing the incidence of infection (seroconversion) as well as reducing the severity of infectious symptoms.[26,27] One would hope that if CMV plays an important role in the development of cardiac allograft vasculopathy the increased use of this agent will likewise diminish the incidence of the vascular disease.

There are several potential directions to take in the development and use of antiviral agents in transplantation. One approach would be to develop antiviral agents that may be extremely toxic long-term but are very effective acutely. These agents could then be utilized to perfuse the donated organ in vitro prior to transplantation. Alternatively, agents previously discarded because of long-term toxicity could be considered in the donor after brain death but prior to organ donation.

An extension of the ever expanding monoclonal antibody field is the development of hybrid molecules which couple specific antibody binding sites to a variety of compounds including cell toxins and isotopes. These hybrid molecules are currently undergoing investigation in a variety of areas including transplantation.[28] One could easily envision a monoclonal antibody directed against specific viral antigens coupled to an antiviral compound for more specific delivery and high concentrations. This technique would be most effective in the treatment of latent viri where numbers of viral copies are relatively smaller than during acute active infection. The obvious problems that would have to be overcome would be among other things, the development of the specific antiviral agent and its coupling to the monoclonal antibody, the choice of the specific receptor target and the method to deliver the hybrid molecule to the virus (intracellular).

The use of newer molecular biology techniques in antiviral therapy has also been suggested. One approach discussed primarily in reference to AIDS therapy would include the synthesis of DNA complementary to the message for an important viral protein. By providing large excesses of this cDNA to the site of viral replication, this viral message would be bound and thus inaccessible for protein transcription.

CONCLUSIONS

Virologic diagnosis and treatment has lagged substantially behind that utilized for other microorganisms. It is only in the last three to five years that substantive advances have been made in diagnostic approaches (owing to hybridoma and molecular biologic technology) and less substantive but significant advances in therapy, specifically for CMV disease. With these new technologies, it is likely that certain post-transplant problems such as cardiac allograft vasculopathy and malignancy and their relationship to viral illness will be better understood. Furthermore, one can anticipate future advances in early diagnosis and potentially new approaches to therapy.

REFERENCES

1. Dummer JS, White LT, Ho M et al. Morbidity of cytomegalovirus infection in recipients of heart or heart-lung transplants who received cyclosporine. J Infect Dis 1985; 152:1182.
2. Smith CB. Cytomegalovirus pneumonia state of the art. Chest 1989; 95(suppl):182S.
3. Bloom JN, Palestine AG. The diagnosis of cytomegalovirus retinitis. Ann Int Med 1988; 109:963.
4. Gonwa TA, Capehart JE, Pilcher JW et al. Cytomegalovirus myocarditis as a cause of cardiac dysfunction in a heart transplant recipient. Transplant 1989; 47:197.
5. Richardson WP, Colvin RB, Cheeseman SH et al. Glomerulopathy associated with cytomegalovirus viremia in renal allografts. N Engl J Med 1981; 305.
6. Grattan MT, Moreno-Cabral EC, Starnes VA et al. Cytomegalovirus infection is associated with cardiac allograft rejection and atherosclerosis. JAMA 1989; 261:3561
7. Hosenpud JD, Chou S, Wagner CR. Cytomegalovirus induced regulation of major histocompatibility complex class I antigen expression in human aortic smooth muscle cells. Transplantation 1991; 52:896.
8. Penn I. Allograft transplant cancer registry. In: DT Purtiilo, ed. Immune Deficiency and Cancer: Epstein-Barr Virus and Lymphoproliferative Malignancies. New York: Plenum Publishing, 1984:281.
9. Cleary ML, Sklar J. Lymphoproliferative disorders in cardiac transplant recipients are multiclonal lymphomas. Lancet 1984; 2:491.
10. Starzl RE, Nalesnik MA, Porter KA et al. Reversibility of lymphomas and lymphoproliferative lesions developing under cyclosporine-steroid therapy. Lancet 1984; 1:583.
11. Tzakis AG, Cooper MH, Dummer JS et al. Transplantation in HIV+ Patients. Transplant 1990;49:354.
12. Degos F, Lugassy C, Degott C et al. Hepatitis B virus and hepatitis B-related viral infectin in renal transplant recipients: A prospective study of 90 patients. Gastroenterology 1988; 94:151.
13. Flagg GL, Silberman H, Takamoto SK et al. Influence of hepatitis B infection on the outcome of renal allotransplantation. Transplant Proc 1987; 19:2155.
14. Colledan M, Grendele M, Gridelli B et al. Long term results after liver transplantation in β and delta hepatitis. Transplant Proc 1989; 21:2421.
15. Dienstag JL. Hepatitis non-A, non-B: C at last. Gastroenterology 1990;99:1177.
16. Read A, Donegan E, Zeldis J et al. Hepatitis C virus (HCV) in patients undergoing liver transplantation. Presented at the XIII International Congress of the Transplantation Society, San Francisco 1990.
17. Chou S. Newer methods for diagnosis of cytomegalovirus infection. Rev Infect Dis 1990; 12(S)7:S727.
18. Kandolf R, Ameis D, Kirschner P et al. In situ detection of enteroviral genomes in myocardial cells by nucleic acid hybridization: an approach to the diagnosis of viral heart disease. Proc Natl Acad Sci USA 1987; 84:6272.
19. Chou S. Differentiation of cytomegalovirus strains by restriction analysis of DNA sequences amplified from clinical specimens. J Infect Dis 1990; 162:738.
20. Chou S, Norman DJ. The influence of donor factors other than serologic status on transmission of cytomegalovirus to transplant recipients. Transplant 1988; 46:89.
21. Wagner CR, Hosenpud JD. Enhanced lymphocyte proliferative responses to donor-specific aortic endothelial cells following influenza vaccine. Transplant Immunology (in press).
22. Meyers JD, Lesczynski J, Zaia JA et al. Prevention of cytomegalovirus infection by cytomegalovirus immunoglobulin after marrow transplatation. Ann Intern Med 1983; 98:442.
23. Hanto DW, Gajl-Peczalska KJ, Balfour HH et al. Acyclovir therapy of Epstein-Barr virus-induced posttransplant lymphoproliferative disease. Trans-

plant Proc 1985; 17:89.

24. Watson FS, O'Connell JB, Amber IJ et al. Treatment of cytomegalovirus pneumonia in heart transplant recipients with 9(1,3-dihydroxy -2-proproxy-methyl)-guanine (DHPG). J Heart Transplant 1988; 7:102.

25. Keay S, Petersen E, Icenogle T et al. Ganciclovir treatment of serious cytomegalovirus infection in heart and heart-lung transplant recipients. Rev Infect Dis 1988; 10(suppl 3):S563.

26. Guillemain R, Garge D, Amrein C et al. Prophylactic use of ganciclovir (DHPG) in heart transplant

recipients (HTR): A preliminary report. Presented at the XIII International Congress of the Transplantation Society, San Francisco 1990.

27. Laske A, Mohacsi P, Gallino A et al. Prophylaxsis with Gancyclovir for cytomegalovirus infection in heart transplantation. Presented at the XIII International Congress of the Transplantation Society, San Francisco 1990.

28. Kirkman RL, Bacha P, Barrett LV et al. Prolongation of cardiac allograft survival in murine recipients treated with a diphtheria toxin-related Interleukin-2 fusion protein. Transplantation 1989; 47:327.

CHAPTER 12

FUTURE IMPROVEMENTS IN IMMUNOSUPPRESSION FOLLOWING CARDIAC TRANSPLANTATION

Dale G. Renlund   Stephanie L. Olsen

R. Douglas Ensley   Michael R. Bristow

INTRODUCTION

Cardiac transplantation has evolved from a fledgling clinical experiment in the late 1960s to an accepted treatment modality in some patients with end-stage cardiac disease.[1] In the past 10 years, the clinical outcome of heart transplantation has dramatically improved, primarily because of improvements in immunosuppressive techniques which include the development of new agents. (Table I)[2] Prior to 1980 (the precyclosporine era), the immunosuppressive therapeutic index (ITI),[3] the ratio of efficacy to toxicity, was extremely low. With cyclosporine-based immunosuppression, the ITI has markedly increased, leading to both improvements in survival and in quality of life.[4] This in turn led to a liberalization of recipient selection criteria[5] and a proliferation of centers offering cardiac transplantation.[6]

Unfortunately, immunosuppression following cardiac transplantation is still far from ideal. Allograft rejection and infection, related to ineffective and inappropriate immunosuppression, respectively, remain the leading causes of death. Also, inadequate immunosuppression from the standpoint of antibody-mediated immunologic injury of coronary vascular endothelium is probably the cause of allograft coronary artery disease, a major impediment to long-term survival following cardiac transplantation.[7] Despite the suppression of cell-mediated allograft rejection, immune-mediated endothelial injury and the reparative events that follow may lead to this chronic form of rejection that manifests as coronary vasculopathy in the cardiac allograft.

In a general sense, in order to further improve immunosuppression in cardiac transplantation, both cell- and antibody-mediated aspects of the immune system

Table 1. Currently Available Immunosuppressive Armamentarium

AGENT	MECHANISM OF ACTION
Cyclosporine	Blocks the secretion of interleukin-2 from helper T lymphocytes, inhibiting the formation of cytotoxic T lymphocytes
Azathioprine	Inhibits purine ring biosynthesis and nucleotide inter-conversions, blocking lymphocyte proliferation
Cyclosphosphamide	An alkylating agent that prevents lymphocyte proliferation by cross-linking DNA
Corticosteroids	Lympholytic, block macrophage inhibitory factor, impairing antigen recognition
Polyclonal antibodies*	Opsonize lymphocytes which are thereafter removed from the circulation by the recipient reticuloendothelial system
Murine monoclonal CD-3antibody (OKT3)	Opsonizes CD-3 positive lymphocytes, immunomodulates lymphocytes, prevents signal transduction of antigen recognition
Vincristine	Prevents lymphocyte proliferation by inhibiting micro-tubular function
Methotrexate	Inhibits purine ring biosynthesis, preventing lympho-cyte proliferation

*Antithymocyte, Antilymphocyte, and Antilymphoblast globulins (ATG, ALG) prepared from sensitized animals (horse, goat, or rabbit). No generally attainable, commercial preparation is available.

need to be more selectively or powerfully inhibited without increasing the side effects associated with over-immunosuppression. In other words, a decreased risk of allograft rejection and coronary artery disease needs to be coupled with a decreased risk of infectious, malignant, and corticosteroid-induced complications. Future improvements in immunosuppression will be considered within the following conceptual framework:

1. Without altering either the intrinsic antigenic potential or stimulus of the allograft or the intrinsic capability of the host immune responses,

2. Decreasing the intrinsic antigenicity of the allograft without intrinsically changing the capability of host immune responses, and

3. Intrinsically altering the response of the recipient's immune system to the allograft

without intrinsically changing the antigenic potential of the allograft.

DECREASED ALLOGRAFT REJECTION WITHOUT ALTERING INTRINSIC ALLOGRAFT ANTIGENICITY OR THE INTRINSIC CAPABILITY OF HOST IMMUNE RESPONSES

Accomplishment of this goal means that the ITI needs to dramatically increase, something that is unlikely with the available immunosuppressive armamentarium (Table 1). New agents have to be discovered, developed, and introduced into clinical practice. These new agents could, alone or in combination with other new agents or with existing agents, more selectively potently interfere with the cascade of events leading to allograft rejection. (Fig. 1)

Several new agents are undergoing or are soon likely to undergo clinical trials in cardiac transplant recipients. (Table 2) Additionally, new immunosuppressive agents will no doubt continue to be discovered through classical or new cellular/molecular biologic screening techniques. Since the mechanisms of action of these new (as well as the current) immunosuppressive agents are heterogeneous, combinations of these agents can easily be imagined that could potently, selectively, and potentially synergistically interrupt the cascade of events leading to allograft rejection.

FK506

FK506 is a macrolide lactone isolated from *Streptomyces tsukubaensis* in 1984.[8-14] While the mechanism of action of FK506 is similar

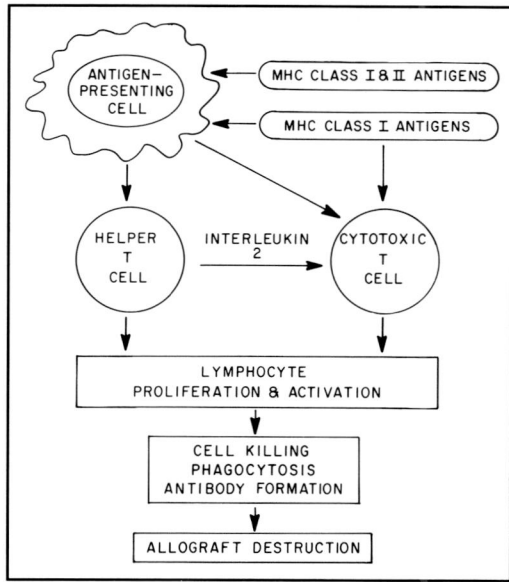

Fig. 1. Cascade of events leading to allograft destruction. Allograft rejection occurs when foreign antigen is processed by antigen-presenting cells and presented to mature helper or cytotoxic T lymphocytes. Processed antigen presented to helper T lymphocytes induces the formation of cytotoxic T lymphocytes by the synthesis and secretion of interleukin-2. Once mature T lymphocytes have recognized foreign antigen, lymphocyte proliferation occurs leading to cell killing, phagocytosis and antibody formation. Left unchecked, allograft destruction ultimately occurs.

to that of cyclosporine, interfering with interleukin-2 production, FK506 appears to be considerably more potent. FK506 inhibits the generation of cytotoxic T cells and the appearance of interleukin-2 receptors on T lymphocytes in human mixed lymphocyte reactions at concentrations 32-100 fold lower than cyclosporine. Animal and human studies have demonstrated the efficacy of FK506 in liver, kidney, and heart transplantation. Ongoing clinical trials will determine whether FK 506 represents a significant advance in immunosuppression.

RS-61443

RS-61443, a morpholinoethylester of mycophenolic acid, is a noncompetitive inhibitor of inosine 5'-monophosphate dehydrogenase and guanosine monophosphate synthetase. Administration of RS-61443 in model systems results in a selective decrease in intracellular guanine nucleotide pools and specific depression of de novo purine biosynthesis.[15,16] With the exception of lymphocytes, all human cells have both a de novo and a salvage pathway for purine biosynthesis. Since lymphocytes only have a de novo pathway, lymphocyte differentiation and proliferation should be specifically inhibited by RS-61443. In animal models of transplantation, RS-61443 has clearly demonstrated efficacy.[17] Current clinical trials in rheumatoid arthritis and in kidney and heart transplantation are ongoing.

RAPAMYCIN

Rapamycin is a macrocyclic triene antibiotic produced by *Streptomyces hygroscopicus*, an actinomycete that was isolated from a soil sample collected from the Vai Atore region of Easter Island.[18,19] Rapamycin is a potent inhibitor of murine thymocyte proliferation[20] and animal studies suggest that rapamycin is 3 - 30 times more potent than cyclosporine.[21] Since rapamycin suppresses interleukin-2 driven or interleukin-4 driven T cell proliferation,[22] one would expect it to act synergistically with either cyclosporine or FK506,[23] although competitive inhibition of the immunosuppressive effects of FK506 has been reported.

TABLE 2. Future Immunosuppressive Agents

AGENT	MECHANISM OF ACTION
FK506	Interferes with the production of interleukin-2 from helper T lymphocytes, blocking the induction of cytotoxic T lymphocytes
RS-61443	Blocks the only pathway, the de novo pathway, in lymphocytes for purine biosynthesis
Rapamycin	Suppresses interleukin-2 and interleukin-4 driven lymphocyte proliferation
Antipan T lymphocyte antibody-Ricin A chain immunoconjugate mono-clonal antibody	Blocks protein synthesis in CD-5 positive lymphocytes by enzymatically cleaving a specific adenosine linkage in ribosomal RNA
OKT4a	Selectively reacts with and depletes CD-4 positive lymphocytes, suppressing the generation of primary cytotoxic responses
Anti-interleukin -2 re-ceptor monoclonal antibody	Inhibits functional interleukin -2 to interleukin 2-receptor interaction

CD-5 RICIN CONJUGATE

Antipan T lymphocyte antibody-ricin A chain immunoconjugate monoclonal antibody is a monoclonal antibody directed at the CD-5 surface antigen of human lymphocytes, present on 99% of mature T lymphocytes, conjugated to a ribosomal inhibitory protein.[24,25] The ribosomal inhibitory protein is obtained from the lectin ricin, which is derived from castor beans. Ricin is composed of two polypeptide chains, A and B chains, linked by a disulfide bond. The cytotoxic action of ricin depends on the internalization of the A chain which occurs only if it is bound to the cell surface membrane. The binding function is provided by the B chain which attaches to cell membranes indiscriminately. When the ricin A chain is coupled to a selective ligand, such as a monoclonal antibody, it can be directed to a target cell population. Once internalized, the ricin A chain blocks protein synthesis by enzymatically cleaving a specific adenosine linkage in ribosomal RNA.

MONOCLONAL ANTIBODIES

The murine monoclonal CD-4 antibody is a murine monoclonal antibody produced in a hybridoma cell line.[26,27] It selectively reacts with CD-4 positive lymphocytes causing depletion of CD-4 positive T lymphocytes, thus completely suppressing the generation of any primary cytotoxic responses.

Anti-interleukin-2 receptor monoclonal antibody is a monoclonal antibody directed against the alpha chain (55 KD) of the interleukin-2 receptor.[28] Interfering with the interleukin-2 receptor/interleukin-2 interaction should inhibit the formation of cytotoxic T lymphocytes. While this drug has been shown to prevent early renal allograft rejection in animals and humans, the results in the treatment of acute allograft rejection are to date less promising.[28]

Given the heterogeneity of the mechanisms of action among the newer and current immunosuppressive agents, one can easily conceive of immunosuppressive agent combinations that could more potently inhibit selective aspects of the rejection cascade when compared to currently used regimens. For instance, since cyclosporine prevents interleukin-2 production and rapamycin inhibits interleukin-2 driven lymphocyte proliferation, cyclosporine coupled with rapamycin should synergistically interfere with helper T lymphocyte-mediated induction of killer T lymphocytes. Furthermore, neither drug would then be needed in near toxic doses. If one is then additionally able to prevent lymphocyte proliferation with the addition of a drug, such as RS-61443, that selectively affects lymphocytes (not granulocytes, not red cell precursors), it does not seem too far-fetched to believe that the risk of rejection and allograft coronary artery disease may be coupled with less infectious, malignant, and corticosteroid complications. Simply stated, it seems very likely that the ITI would dramatically increase. Of course, carefully controlled clinical trials will be needed to document safety and efficacy of individual agents and agents used in combinations.

DECREASED ALLOGRAFT REJECTION BY DECREASING INTRINSIC ALLOGRAFT ANTIGENICITY WITHOUT ALTERING THE INTRINSIC CAPABILITY OF HOST IMMUNE RESPONSES

If the antigenic stimulus of the cardiac allograft could be decreased, the vigor of the recipient's immune response would likely decrease, which, in turn, would decrease the amount of immunosuppression required to maintain allograft function. Again, the ITI would dramatically increase. The notion of decreasing the antigenicity of a cardiac allograft dates to the beginning of clinical cardiac transplantation when irradiation of the allograft was performed in many of the early transplant procedures. The impetus for the attempts at reducing the antigenic load of the allograft stems from reports that certain cells in the allograft are more antigenically potent than others. Allograft dendritic cells and passenger leukocytes importantly contribute to the antigenicity of the allograft since long-surviving major histocompatibility complex

(MHC) incompatible rat kidney grafts, when retransplanted from a primary to a secondary recipient of the same genotype, do not elicit strong primary T-dependent alloimmunity in the secondary recipient.[29] Thus, while chronic immunosuppression is required for graft survival in the primary recipient, chronic immunosuppression is not needed in the secondary recipient. Furthermore, strong immunogenicity can be restored by injecting dendritic cells of primary donor origin at the time of retransplantation.[30] A further suggestion of the role of dendritic cells was shown when kidneys subjected to essential fatty acid deficiency, and thus depleted of interstitial macrophages, survived and functioned when transplanted across a major histocompatibility antigen barrier in the absence of immunosuppression of the recipient, whereas control allografts were promptly rejected.[31] These experiments suggest that in the absence of allograft dendritic cells and passenger leukocytes, the propensity of a recipient to reject is decreased. They also raise the intriguing possibility that if antigen recognition is blocked until the allograft dendritic cells and passenger leukocytes are cleared, the vigor of the recipient's immune response would be decreased without having intrinsically altered the capabilities of the recipient's immune system.[3]

Since OKT3 blocks T lymphocyte receptor-mediated signal transduction of antigen recognition, OKT3 was introduced into early rejection prophylaxis protocols following cardiac transplantation in the hopes of blocking the recognition of the highly antigenic dendritic cells and passenger leukocytes until they were cleared from the allograft. Two trials have given indirect evidence supporting the notion that early, aggressive rejection prophylaxis leads to more complete allograft tolerance. In the first study, comparing OKT3-based and equine antithymocyte globulin (ATG)-based early rejection prophylaxis, the OKT3-based protocol decreased the risk of rejection when compared to the ATG-based protocol.[32] The OKT3 group averaged 32% fewer episodes of rejection/patient during the first six months following transplantation despite similar six month cumulative cyclosporine and azathioprine doses and 37% less corticosteroid administration. Importantly, more patients in the OKT3 group successfully discontinued maintenance corticosteroids (88% versus 46%). Despite being less immunosuppressed, the OKT3-treated patients had less propensity to reject later, as evidenced by a 68% decrease in rejection frequency when compared with the ATG-based patients during the interval between 6 and 12 months, an interval well beyond the period during which the early rejection prophylaxis protocols differed. Of note, most randomized studies of OKT3 in renal transplantation similarly suggest that the propensity to develop allograft rejection late is decreased following prophylactic OKT3 administration.

In the second study, a decreased propensity to reject well beyond the time of the early rejection prophylaxis protocols was seen with a longer course of OKT3 when comparing a 14-day to 10-day OKT3 administration.[33] During the interval between 3 and 6 months, the 14-day OKT3-based patients rejected 42% less than the 10-day OKT3-based patients.

While these latter two studies are in no way conclusive, they do suggest that aggressive early rejection prophylaxis may affect a recipient's long-term propensity to reject. The most plausible explanation is that blockade of antigen recognition early following transplantation decreases the antigenic potential of the allograft, resulting in a less vigorous recipient immune response.

OKT3 is not ideally suited to prolonged administration and by itself, therefore, is unable to test the underlying hypothesis that blockade of antigen recognition until the highly antigenic dendritic cells and passenger leukocytes are cleared from the allograft results in a decreased need for chronic immunosuppression. Although the hypothesis is not proven, it is certainly not disproven. To test the hypothesis one would require either an agent that specifically blocks antigen recognition safely forgreater than one month or an agent with which the allograft can be pretreated to hasten the loss of the dendritic cells and passenger leukocytes.

DECREASED ALLOGRAFT REJECTION BY ALTERING INTRINSIC HOST IMMUNE RESPONSES WITHOUT ALTERING THE INTRINSIC ANTIGENICITY OF THE ALLOGRAFT

The ultimate goal of immunosuppression following cardiac transplantation is that there be no need for any, i.e., the induction of completely selective, permanent tolerance of donor antigens by the recipient's immune system. In general, allograft tolerance, a reduction in the immunocompetence of the recipient lymphocyte pool toward donor antigens, could come about in three ways.[34] First, the number of cells capable of responding to donor antigens could be decreased, second, a reduction in the degree to which each cell is stimulated although the number of cells capable of responding to donor antigens remains unchanged, and finally, by having both an unchanged number and capability to respond to the antigenic stimuli, but with activation impeded by regulatory cells within the lymphoid population, i.e., specific suppressor cells.

Clonal depletion, clonal anergy, and possibly several other mechanisms within the recipient could enable decreased responsiveness to specific donor antigens, thus making immunosuppressive therapy unnecessary or at least markedly decreased in the long-term. The desirability of this goal has generated intensive investigations over the years that are leading to successful strategies in animal models. Many recent reports have demonstrated the induction of tolerance by using some combination of donor antigens coupled with other therapy (such as the administration of a CD-4 monoclonal antibody) prior to transplantation.[35,36] These studies demonstrate that the tolerance induction is possible under certain experimental conditions. It seems likely that similarly conducted protocols may one day be applicable to human cardiac transplantation.

CONCLUSION

In summary, future improvements in immunosuppression may result from: (1) the introduction of newer, more potent or more selective immunosuppressive agents, (2) alteration of the intrinsic antigenicity of the allograft, or from (3) alteration of the intrinsic responses of the recipient's immune system to the allograft. While these three circumstances can be considered separately, it is likely that improvement in immunosuppression will come about, to some extent at least, as a result of all three. Finally, the hope that immunosuppression will improve following cardiac transplantation in the years to come is not only realistic and but highly likely.

REFERENCES

1. Medicare program; criteria for medicare coverage of heart transplants. Fed Regist 1986; 51:37164-37170.
2. Woodley SL, Renlund DG, O'Connell JB, Bristow MR. Immunosuppression following cardiac transplantation. Cardiology Clinics 1990; 8:83-96.
3. Renlund DG, O'Connell JB, Bristow MR. Strategies of immunosuppression in cardiac transplantation. Seminars in thoracic and cardiovascular surgery 1990; 2:181-188.
4. Oyer E, Stinson EB, Jamieson SW, Hunt SA, Perlroth M, Billingham M, Shumway NE. Cyclosporine in cardiac transplantation: A 2 1/2 year follow-up. Transplant Proc 1983; 15:2546-2552.
5. Olsen SL, O'Connell JB. Changing spectrum of candidacy for cardiac transplantation. Heart Failure 1989; 5:228-235.
6. Ontkean M, Hosenpud JD. Emergence of routine survival following orthotopic cardiac transplantation. Heart Failure 1989; 5:219-227.
7. Ratkovec RM, Wray RB, Renlund DG et al. Influence of corticosteroid-free maintenance immunosuppression on allograft coronary artery disease following cardiac transplantation. J Thorac Cardiovasc Surg 1190; 100:6-12.
8. Nalesnik MA, Todo S, Murase N. Toxicology of FK-506 in the lewis rat. Transplant Proc 1989; 19:89-92.
9. Ochiai T, Hamaguchi K, Isono KK. Histopathologic studies in renal transplant recipient dogs receiving treatment with FK506. Transplant Proc 1987; 19:93-97.
10. Thiru S, Collier DStJ, Calne R. Pathological studies in canine and baboon renal allograft recipients immunosuppressed with FK506. Transplant Proc 1987; 19:98-99.
11. Collier DStJ, Calne R, Thiru S. FK-506 in experimental renal allografts. Transplant Proc 1987; 19:3975-3977.
12. Thomson AW, Stephen ME, Woo J, Hasan NU, Whiting PH. Immunosuppressive activity, T-cell subset analysis, and acute toxicity of FK506 in rats. Transplant Proc 1989; 21:1048-1049.
13. Morimoto T, Yamada F, Kobayashi Tet al. Blood levels of FK506 after intramuscular and intravenous administration in dogs. Transplant Proc 1989; 21:1059-1063.
14. Yokota KK, Takishima T, Sato K. Comparative studies of FK506 and cyclosporine in canine orthotopic hepatic allograft survival. Transplant Proc 1989; 21:1066-1068.
15. Franklin TJ, Cook JM. The inhibition of nucleic acid synthesis by mycophenolic acid. Biochem J 1969; 113:515-524.
16. Platz KP, Sollinger HW, Hullett DA, Eckhoff DE, Eugui EM, Allison AC. RS-61443- A new, potent immunosuppressive agent. Transplantation 1991; 51:27-31.
17. Morris RE, Grant HE, Eugui EM, Allison AC. Prolongation of rat heart allograft survival by RS 61443. Surg Forum 1989; 40:337-338.
18. Vezina C, Kudelsi A, Sehgal SN. Rapamycin (AY-22989), a new antifungal antibiotic. I. Taxonomy of the producing streptomycete and isolation of the active principle. J Antibiotics 1975; 28:721-732.
19. Sehgal SN, Baker H, Vezina C. Rapamycin (AY-22,989), a new antifungal antibiotic. II. Fermentation, isolation and characterization. J Antibiotics 1975; 28:727-732.
20. Adams LM, Warner LW, Baeder WL, Sehgal SN, Chang JY. Immunosuppressive activity of rapamycin vs. cyclosporin A. J Cell Biol 1989; 109(number 4, part II):163a.
21. Stepkowski SM, Chen H, Daloze P, Kahan BD. Rapamycin, a potent immunosuppressive drug for vascularized heart, kidney, and small bowel transplantation in the rat. Transplant 1990; 51:22-26.
22. Dumont FJ, Melino MR, Staruch MJ, Koprak SL, Fischer PA, Sigal NH. The immunosuppressive macrolides FK506 and rapamycin act as reciprocal antagonists in murine T cells. J Immunol 1990; 144:1418-1424.
23. Kahan BD, Gibbons S, Tejpal N, Stepkowski SM, Chou T-C. Synergistic interactions of cyclosporine and rapamycin to inhibit immune performances of normal human peripheral blood lymphocytes in vitro. Transplantation 1991; 51:232-239.
24. Olsnes S, Refsnes K, Pihl A. Mechanism or action of the toxic lectins abrin and ricin. Nature 1974; 249:627-631.
25. Kernan NA, Knowles RW, Burns MJ et al. Specific inhibition of in vitro lymphocyte transformation by an anti-pan T cell (gp67) ricin A chain immunoconjugate. J Immunol 1984; 133:137-146.
26. Weyand CM, Goronzy J, Swarztrauber, Fathman CG. Immunosuppression by anti-CD4 treatment in vivo. Transplantation 1989; 47:1034-1038.
27. Cole JA, McCarthy SA, Rees MA, Sharrow SO, Singer A. Cell surface comodulation of CD4 and T cell receptor by anti-CD4 monoclonal antibody. J Immunol 1989; 143:397-402.

28. Cantarovich D, Le Mauff B, Hourmant M et al. Anti-interleukin 2 receptor monoclonal antibody in the treatment of ongoing acute rejection episodes of human kidney graft- A pilot study. Transplantation 1989; 47:454-457.

29. Hart DNJ, Winearls CG, Fabre JW. Graft adaptation: Studies on possible mechanisms in long surviving rat renal allografts. Transplantation 1980; 30:73-78.

30. Lechler RI, Batchelor JR. Restoration of immunogenicity to passenger cell-depleted kidney allografts by the addition of donor strain dendritic cells. J Exp Med 1982; 155:31-41.

31. Schreiner GF, Flye W, Brunt E, Korber K, Lefkowith JB. Essential fatty acid depletion of renal allografts and prevention of rejection. Science 1988; 240:1032-1033.

32. Renlund DG, O'Connell JB, Gilbert EM. A prospective comparison of murine monoclonal CD-3 antibody-based and equine antithymocyte globulin-based rejection prophylaxis in cardiac transplantation: Decreased rejection and less corticosteroid use with OKT3. Transplantation 1989; 47:599-605.

33. Hegewald MG, O'Connell JB, Renlund DG. OKT3 monoclonal antibody given for 10 versus 14 days as immunosuppression prophylaxis in cardiac transplantation. J Heart Transplant 1989; 8:303-310.

34. Nossal GJV. Immunologic tolerance. In: Paul WE, ed. Fundamental Immunology. 2nd ed. New York: Raven Press,1989:571-586.

35. Wood KJ, Morris PJ. Avenues for acquired immune tolerance. Semin Thorac Cardiovasc Surg 1990; 2:189-197.

36. Benjamin RJ, Waldmann H. Induction of tolerance by monoclonal antibody therapy. Nature 1986; 320:449-451.

CHAPTER 13

NOVEL APPROACHES TO IMMUNOSUPPRESSION: PEPTIDES, ADHESION MOLECULES AND TOLERANCE

Daniel R. Salomon

The recent development of multiple new immunosuppressive drugs is clearly exciting. However, in the view of cellular immunology the majority of these new drugs remain essentially nonspecific inhibitors of T cell activation. In the present chapter I will review two developments in our understanding of T cell activation at the molecular level that promise novel applications to immunosuppression in the next decade.

    1) Antigen presentation and peptides
    2) Adhesion molecules

ANTIGEN PRESENTATION AND PEPTIDES

The recognition of foreign or donor HLA antigens by highly specific receptors expressed on the T cell surface remains the critical control element for the immune response in transplantation. However, these antigens must be presented to the T cell in a very special way for the process to work.[1,2] The donor HLA antigens must be presented in the context of the patient's own HLA molecules — a process called *restriction*. This is accomplished by *antigen processing* during which a relatively large foreign HLA molecule is taken up by the patient's cell and broken down into several key fragments called *peptides*. In fact, it appears that these peptides may be only 9 to 12 amino acids long. As shown in Figure 1, the structure of the HLA molecule creates a pocket on its outer surface which is called the *antigen-binding groove*.[3] We now understand that while still inside the cell, the selected foreign peptides are placed in the antigen-binding groove of the patient's own HLA molecules. (Fig. 2) The molecule is then transported to the cell surface where the T cell can recognize the foreign peptide literally "in the arms" of the patient's own HLA molecule. In fact, this presentation pathway is the same for viral, bacterial, chemical and tumor antigens.

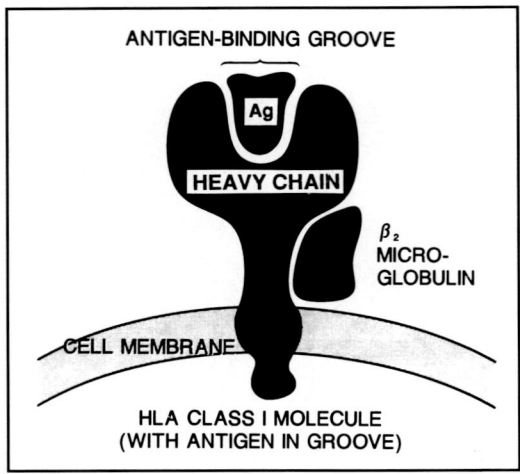

Fig. 1. Class I HLA molecule showing the antigenic peptide carried in the antigen-binding groove on its upper surface.

It is tempting to simplify matters by concluding that the HLA molecules normally expressed on the cell surfaces of all tissues have empty antigen-binding grooves which are just waiting for the chance to present a foreign peptide. However, we now know that peptides derived from inside the patient's own cell normally occupy the grooves. These *endogenous* or *self-peptides* are specific for the patient's HLA molecules and play a critical role in the development of the adult immune system by allowing us to distinguish self antigens from foreign ones.[3,4] Therefore, our current concept of the HLA system as a unique "signature" for the individual must now also include these self-peptides normally occupying the antigen-binding grooves. (Fig. 2)

The clinical implications of these two concepts are as follows. First, T cells recognize small peptide fragments of the donor

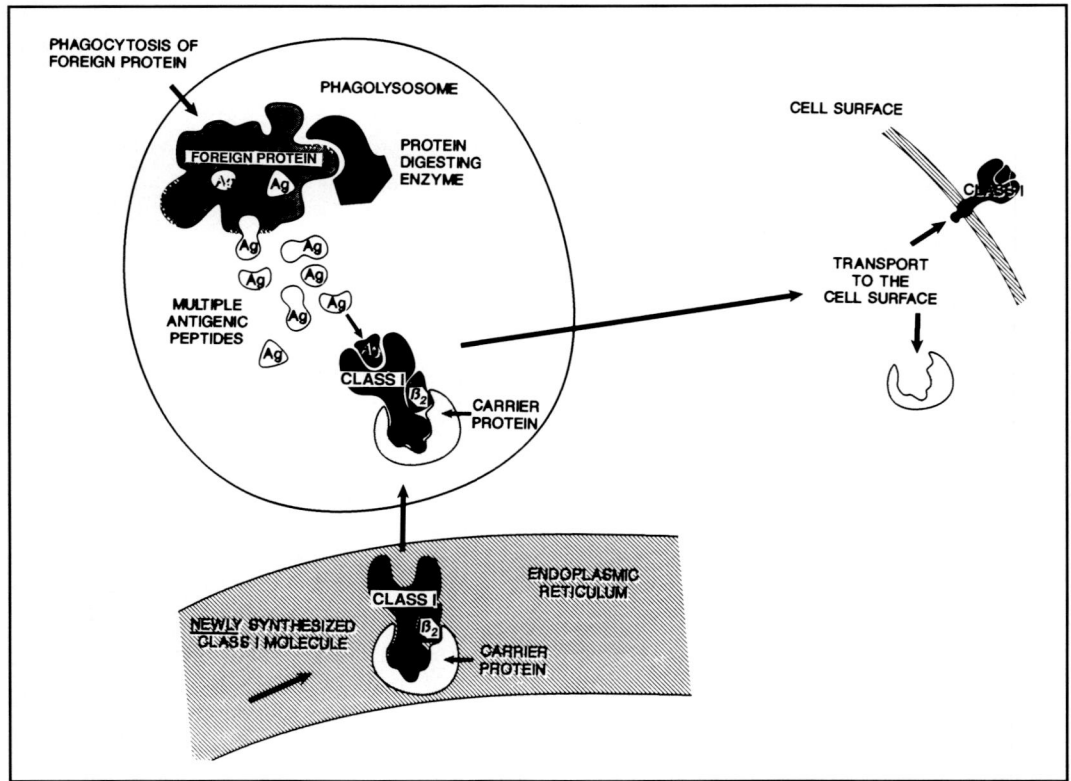

Fig. 2. Diagram of how a foreign peptide is digested in the phagolysosome into multiple small antigenic peptides. A newly synthesized class I HLA molecule is transported "empty" from the endoplasmic reticulum into the phagolysosome and selects only the antigenic peptides that are complementary to the structure of its binding groove. Finally, the "loaded" class I molecule is transported to the cell surface for antigen presentation. This entire process is often called antigen processing and presentation.

HLA molecule not the entire molecule. Thus, if we could determine the sequence of the peptides we could easily reproduce them in a laboratory. These peptides could be infused into patients to confuse T cells or block T cell activation by competing for binding with the peptides in the HLA grooves. (Fig. 3) Maybe they could be altered slightly so that they would not be recognized by the T cell receptor but they could still bind and displace the donor peptides in the grooves. What if we made antibodies against the peptides - would they bind and prevent T cell recognition? Could we use them as "vaccines"? Remember that these peptides are highly specific for the donor HLA molecules and, thus, theoreti-

cally these immunosuppressive strategies would have no effect on the immune response to viral, bacterial or tumor antigens. If the patient's cells must first process and then present these foreign peptides perhaps we can develop drugs that inhibit this event. In fact, a new drug called Brefeldin A may be the first such example.[5] Finally, if the self-peptides described above are unique to specific HLA molecules it follows that the patient's T cells may also recognize the donor as foreign by direct recognition of the donor HLA molecules presenting their self-peptides. Therefore, the same strategies considered above for the processed foreign peptides are also applicable to these self-peptides. Would it be pos-

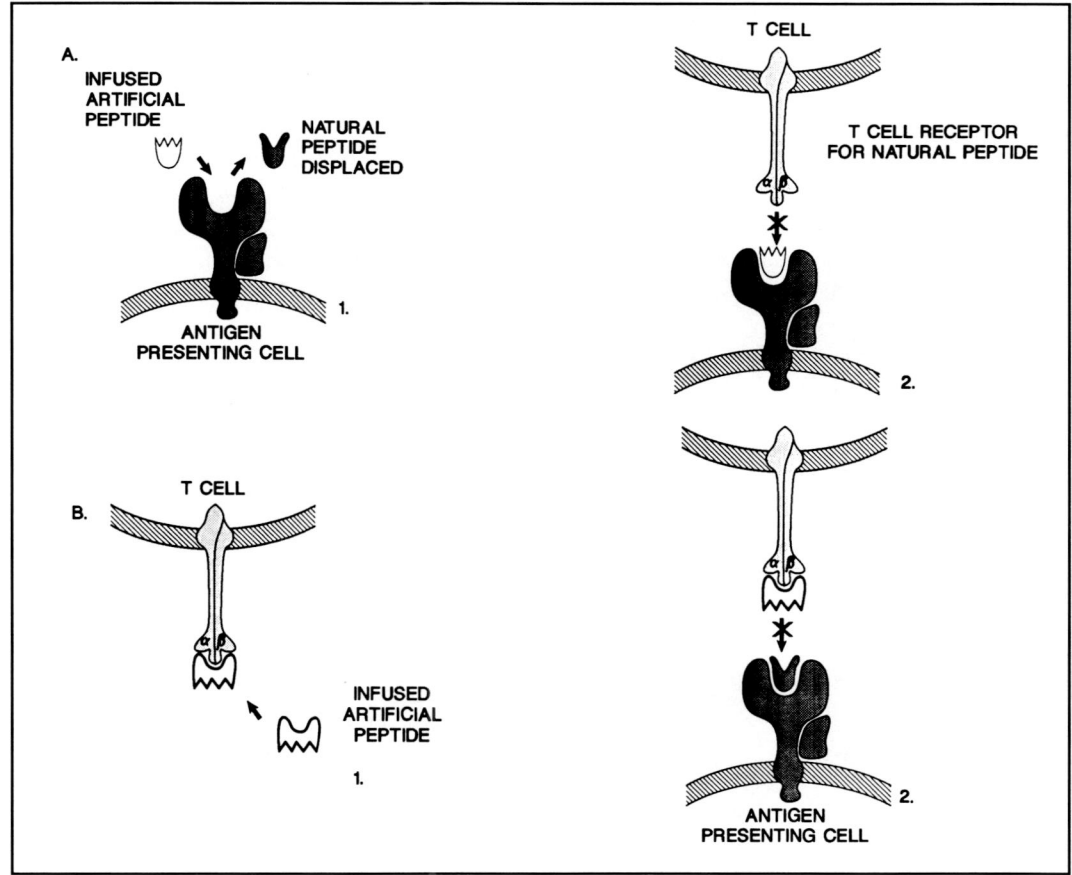

Fig. 3. Synthesized antigenic peptides can be used to block the immune response in at least two ways. (1.) A peptide engineered to mimic the class I binding groove site but with a different exterior surface competes the natural peptide out of the groove. The t cell does not recognize the engineered antigen's surface and ignores it. (2.) A peptide is engineered to mimic the exterior surface of the natural peptide -—the t cell binding site -—and binds to the t cells. However, it cannot be bound by the class I molecule. The t cell cannot find the antigen presenting cell and, thus, is effectively blocked.

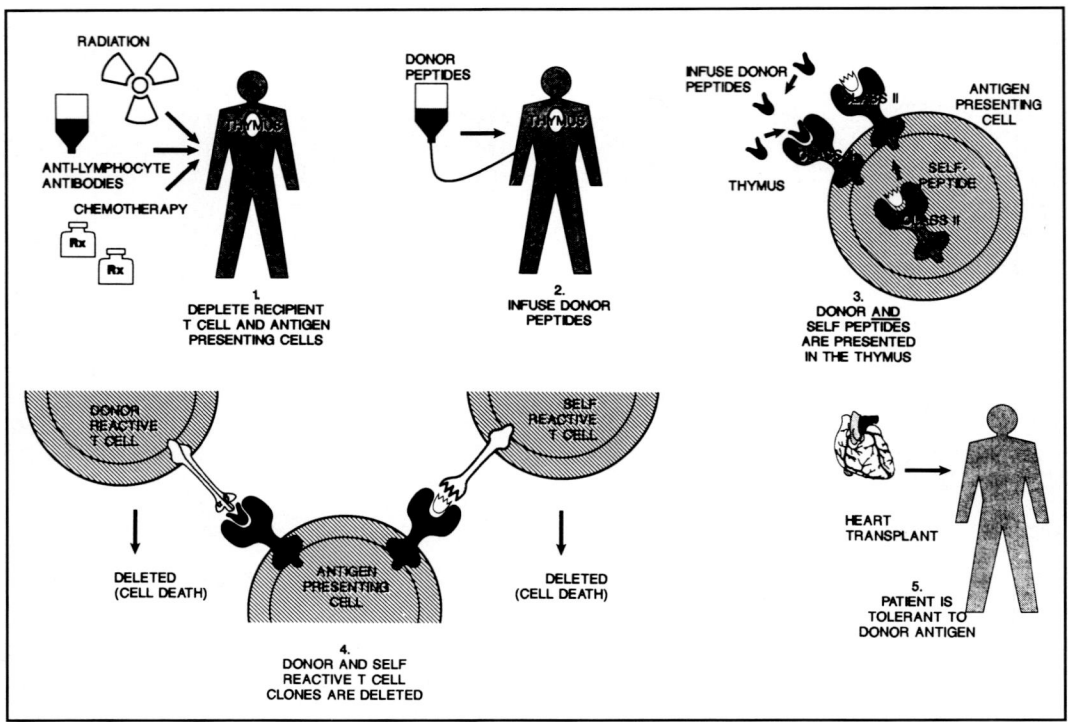

Fig. 4. Donor specific tolerance can be created by first destroying the patient's immune system and then loading the antigen presenting cells with donor peptide. When the new T cells come to the thymus for selection they will see the donor peptide as "self" and be deleted.

sible to trick the patient's immune system into thinking that the donor was self? We think that the definition of self is based on the recognition of self-peptides in HLA molecules by early T cell progenitors in the thymus. Therefore, it may be possible to re-educate the adult T cell system by first destroying the mature circulating T cells and then exposing the early T cell progenitors to donor self-peptides. (Fig. 4)

ADHESION MOLECULES AND T CELL ACTIVATION

The recognition of foreign antigen by the T cell receptor described above is a physical event which requires the binding of the T cell receptor to the foreign peptides displayed on the HLA surfaces. It turns out that the affinity of the T cell receptor is not high enough to fully accomplish this critical binding step. Therefore, a simplistic view of adhesion molecules describes them as necessary coparticipants for stable binding of T cells to

antigen-presenting cells or to their intended targets, e.g., a transplanted donor cell during rejection. The CD4 (helper T cells) and CD8 (killer T cells) molecules specifically bind HLA molecules to facilitate T cell recognition of peptide antigens displayed in the grooves. Monoclonal antibodies directed against these adhesion molecules can specifically block otherwise fully functional T cells.

However, we now understand that another large group of adhesion molecules called *integrins* are critical players in the immune response.[6] There are at least three families of integrins expressed by lymphocytes, monocytes, macrophages and platelets. (Fig. 5) They are up-regulated in both numbers and activity (binding affinity) when cells are activated. One integrin family is primarily on lymphocytes and act as receptors for molecules expressed by antigen presenting cells.[7] Obviously, these integrins are involved in stabilizing T cell binding for antigen recognition. However, what is exciting is that these integrins are also required to signal a T cell for activation. In other words, without the *costimulation* of the integrin molecule, the T cell will not activate despite recognition of its specific target antigen!

Another function of the integrins is to bind to extracellular matrix (ECM) proteins such as fibronectin, vitronectin, collagen and laminin. The ECM proteins are the structural components of the basement membranes and interstitial spaces. Therefore, these integrins allow lymphocytes and macrophages to cross the vascular basement membranes and enter the interstitial spaces where transplantation rejection occurs. The exposure of these ECM proteins due to various forms of tissue or vascular injury or inflammation plays an important role in the immune response. In fact, these ECM proteins can also serve as costimulatory signals for T cell activation by binding to the integrins.

Finally, the integrins can also recognize another new class of molecules called vascular or endothelial cell adhesion molecules (VCAMs or ENCAMs). These molecules are also up-regulated on endothelial cell surfaces when tissue injury occurs, e.g., rejection or with viral infections. Thus, the binding of lymphocyte integrins to these VCAMs is a means of getting cells to a specific site such as the transplanted organ and this process is called *homing*.

Some of the clinical implications of the integrins are obvious. (Fig. 6) Blocking the critical costimulatory signal required for T cell activation would be a powerful immunosuppressive strategy. Similarly, preventing lymphocytes from homing to transplanted organs or blocking their movement into the interstitial space would prevent rejection despite the circulation of mature, even activated T cells looking for the foreign tissue. Antibody against the integrin molecules would be one blocking strategy while another would be to use synthetic peptides which have now been identified to mimic the ECM proteins binding sites for integrins and prevent cell adhesion. In fact, clinical trials of monoclonal antibodies against certain integrins are just beginning. If donor antigen must first be taken up by the patient's cells for presentation as peptides (see above), then it is possible that blocking the integrin binding step might prevent the

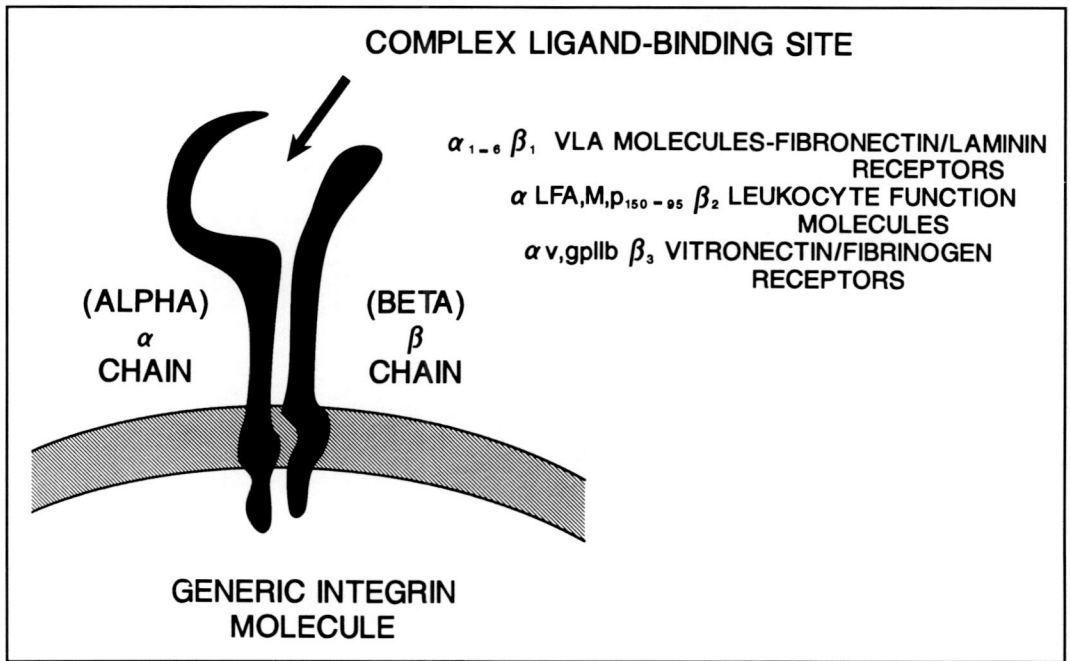

COMPLEX LIGAND-BINDING SITE

$\alpha_{1-6} \beta_1$ VLA MOLECULES-FIBRONECTIN/LAMININ RECEPTORS
α LFA,M,p$_{150-95}$ β_2 LEUKOCYTE FUNCTION MOLECULES
α v,gpIIb β_3 VITRONECTIN/FIBRINOGEN RECEPTORS

(ALPHA)
α
CHAIN

(BETA)
β
CHAIN

GENERIC INTEGRIN MOLECULE

Fig. 5 . *General integrin molecule structure simplified. More recently three additional beta chains have been found and more complex combinations of alpha/beta chains have been described.*

patient's immune system from even knowing a transplant had occurred! This would be exciting enough but another set of observations suggest that integrins might be manipulated to produce tolerance. (Fig. 7)[8] In one experimental system if a T cell recognizes its antigen and receives the integrin signal it is activated normally. In contrast, if the same T cell recognizes the antigen but the integrin signal is blocked, the T cell is not activated as noted above. However, the key observation is that this T cell cannot be activated again in the future even when the antigen is presented and the integrin signal available! In other words, the T cell is now unresponsive to its intended target antigen despite a perfectly functional T cell receptor. This is called *anergy* and is one mechanism for the production of tolerance. Finally, it is likely that the integrins are also involved in the thymus during the development of the adult T cell system alluded to in the previous section on peptide

antigen presentation. Perhaps stimulating the T cell progenitors with donor peptides while manipulating the integrin signal with antibody might further the goal of tricking the patient into accepting the donor as self.

SUMMARY

I have described our current understanding of two fundamental aspects of T cell activation. First, the recognition of self and foreign antigen involves unique peptide fragments processed and then presented in the antigen-binding groove of the HLA molecules. Second, the activation of the T cell requires stable binding plus the costimulatory signals provided by a new class of adhesion molecules called integrins. The role of the integrins in directing lymphocytes to specific sites and the possibility that T cells may become antigen unresponsive (tolerant) if the integrin signals are blocked was also discussed. In fact,

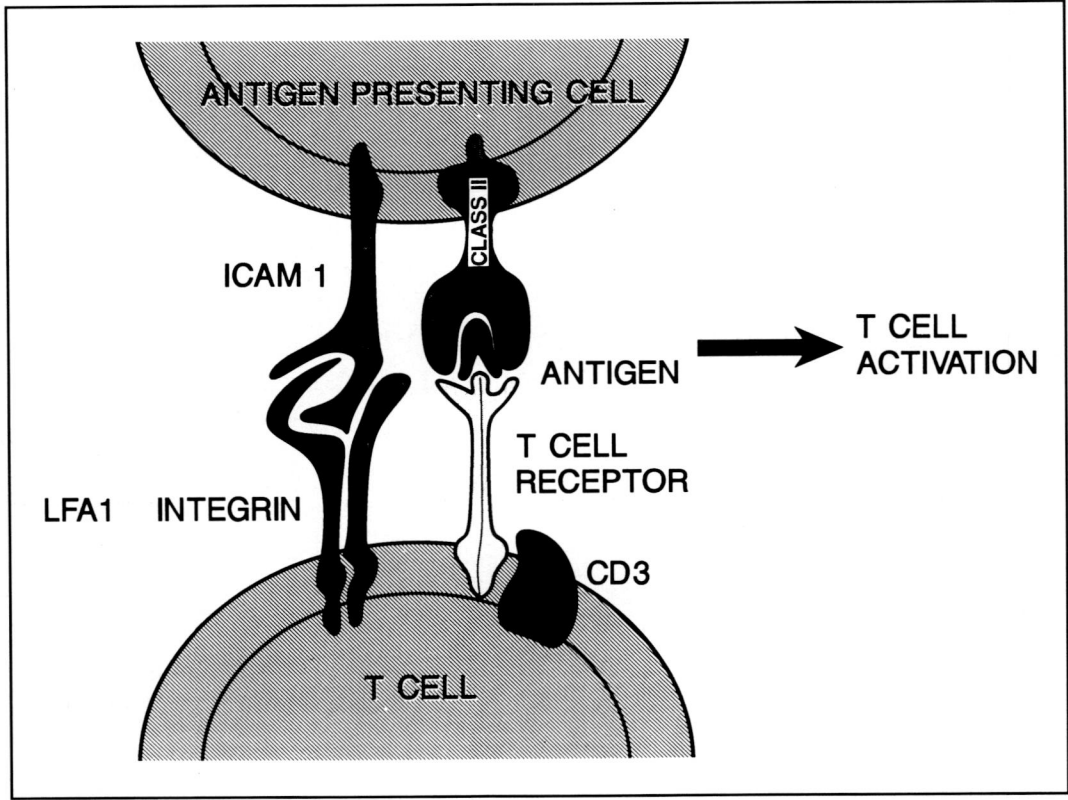

Fig. 6. Simultaneous T cell signalling with both the T cell receptor/CD3 complex and the engaged LFA-1 integrin molecule results in T cell activation. This is a classic model of costimulation.

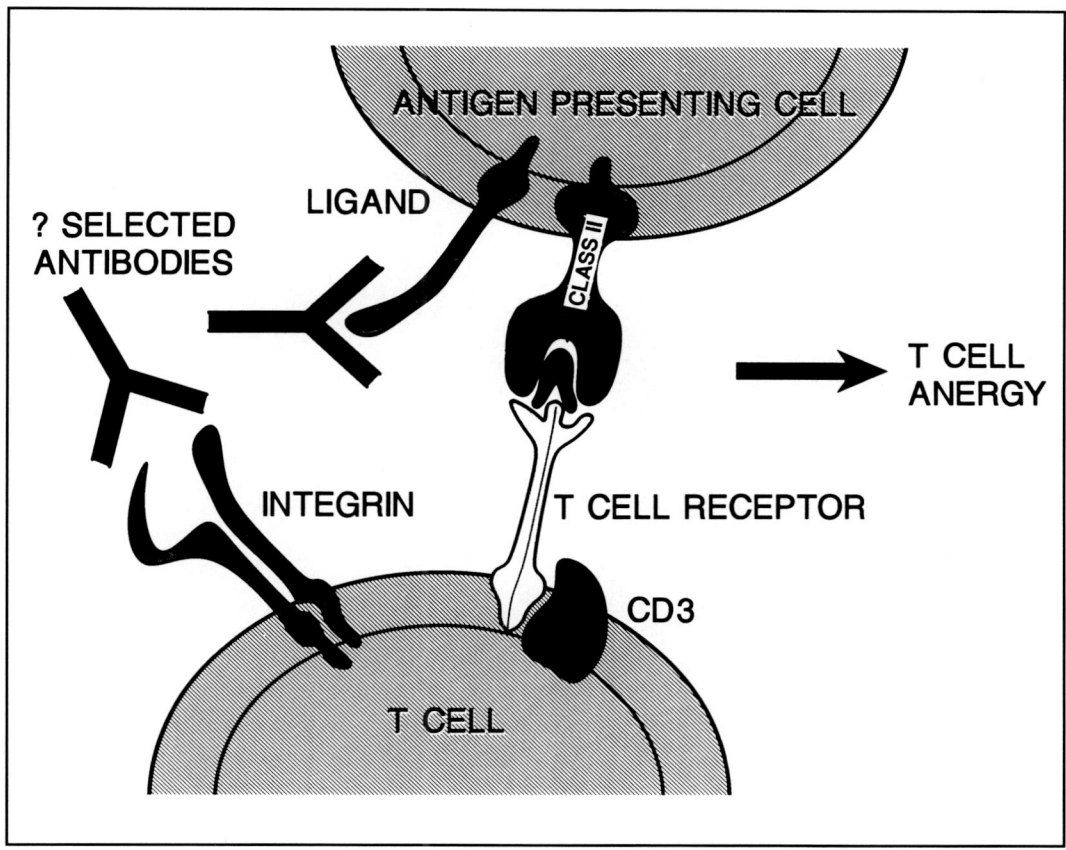

Fig. 7. Theoretically, if the costimulatory signal provided by the integrin molecule is blocked by either antibody to the integrin molecule or its ligand, the T cell will not be activated and might even become anergic (unresponsive) to the donor antigen. The former has already been demonstrated in several models. The latter remains theoretical.

both these aspects of T cell activation are related in that each reveals strategies for specifically altering the nature of the immune response to the transplanted organ. It is highly probable that these reagents will soon be used to significantly improve our ability to prevent and treat transplant rejection. If tolerance can be achieved by these methods in the next decade, the clinical practice of transplanation will be revolutionized.

REFERENCES

1. Delovitch TL, Semple JW, Phillips ML. Influence of antigen processing on immune responsiveness. Immunology Today 1988; 9:216-217.
2. Parham P. Peptide feeding and cellular cookery. Nature 1990; 346:793-795.
3. Sinha AA., Lopez MT, McDevitt HO. Autoimmune diseases: The failure of self tolerance. Science1990; 248:1380-1388.
4. Blackman M, Kappler J, Marrack P. The role of the T cell receptor in positive and negative selection of developing T cells. Science 1990; 248:1335-1341.
5. Chen BP, Madrigal A, Parham P. Cytotoxic T cell recognition of an endogenous class I HLA peptide presented by a class II HLA molecule. Journal of Experimental Medicine 1990; 172:779-788.
6 Springer TA. Adhesion receptors of the immune system. Nature 1990; 346:425-434.
7. Shimuzu Y, vanSeventer GA, Horgan KJ, Shaw S. Roles of adhesion molecules in T cell recognition: Fundamental similarities between four integrins on resting human T cells in expression, binding and costimulation. Immunological Reviews1990; 114:109-143.
8. Schwartz RH. A cell culture model for T lymphocyte clonal anergy. Science 1990; 248:1349-1356.

CHAPTER 14

NEONATAL HEART TRANSPLANTATION: INDICATIONS AND RESULTS

Mario Chiavarelli

Leonard L. Bailey

Heart transplantation has proven to be effective therapy over a broad age span, mainly for treatment of end-stage heart disease which is characterized by nonviable myocardium.

Most of the babies born with complex congenital heart disease have a healthy structural myocardium initially, and they do not fulfill the criteria for end-stage heart disease. The combination of lesions, however, requires multiple palliative operations with significant early mortality. An occasional patient will have long-lasting benefit, but a very large number are lost to operative mortality and natural attrition during and after serial palliative efforts. Therefore, neonatal heart transplantation has been offered as a viable option for treatment of incurable congenital heart anomalies at Loma Linda University Medical Center since November 1985.

Outcome of a therapeutic modality is best evaluated in terms of the time-related benefit, and death is the most unequivocal end-point used to compare results after different forms of treatment for otherwise fatal conditions. Therefore, outcome should be evaluated on the basis of long-term results and actuarial survival rates.

Within this chapter, we will limit discussion to cardiac transplantation as it applies to structural heart disease treated during the first 30 days of life, without including patients with cardiomyopathy and tumors.

ACCEPTED INDICATIONS FOR NEONATAL HEART TRANSPLANTATION

Of the 25,000-30,000 babies born each year in North America with congenital heart disease, perhaps as many as 10% have malformations that preclude corrective surgery.

Hypoplastic left heart syndrome

Newborns with HLHS make up one large category that fits the description of incurable congenital heart disease, and there is no doubt that neonatal transplantation offers better results than staged palliation toward a Fontan procedure. Even in the best hands[1] results with the Norwood procedure have not been encouraging. Out of 200 hundred patients undergoing the first stage reconstruction 17% died during the first postoperative day, and only 62% were discharged from the hospital. Between 1 and 18 months from the initial procedure 30% of the surviving patients required further intervention including shunt revision, arch reconstruction, enlargement of the atrial septal defect, pulmonary artery angioplasty, tricuspid valve procedures, bidirectional cavopulmonary anastomosis or heart transplantation (3 patients). These interim procedures accounted for further loss of patients and lead to an 18-month actuarial survival of 48%. (Fig. 1) Data on the number of survivors that were considered candidates for a Fontan procedure were not provided. Outcome following the Fontan procedure for HLHS is also disturbing; actuarial survival in 74 patients was 75% at 1 month and 60% at 12 months.[2]

Univentricular atrioventricular connection with discordant ventriculo-arterial connection

This diagnosis includes tricuspid atresia and double inlet ventricle associated with transposition of the great arteries and dominant left ventricle. Conventional surgery in this set of lesions is attended with poor long-term survival.[3] Twenty-two infants undergoing pulmonary artery banding and arch reconstruction either died or developed subaortic stenosis within three years of age, and only 9% survived more definitive palliation. Thirty-three patients requiring isolated pulmonary artery banding in infancy showed a five-year actuarial survival free of subaortic stenosis of 57% and fulfilled criteria for a Fontan procedure.

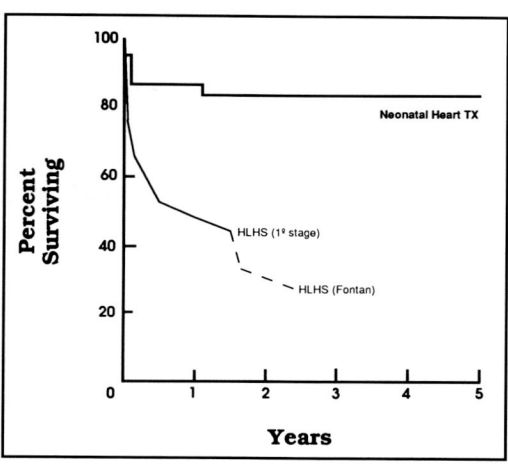

Fig. 1. Actuarial curves at five years of follow-up for the neonatal heart transplant population at Loma Linda University (n=52), and actuarial survival after palliation of hypoplastic left heart syndrome (n=200) at The Children's Hospital of Philadelphia.[1] Results of the Fontan procedure (n=74, dashed curve) for hypoplastic left heart syndrome at the same Institution[2] have been arbitrarily plotted with the first-stage curve, but they refer to a different pool of patients.

Double inlet ventricle

Twenty-nine percent of 191 infants with double inlet ventricle were not potential candidates for a Fontan procedure at presentation, and despite palliative efforts, only 28% of them were alive at one year of age.[4] Among the remaining infants, who were potentially suitable for more definitive palliation initially, actuarial survival was 67% at one year, and unexplained sudden death occurred in 10% of the patients before four years of age. (Fig. 2)

Pulmonary atresia and intact ventricular septum

Infants with PA-IVS have had poor long-term results in the past with an actuarial survival of about 50% at five years and 25% at 10 years. That outcome would qualify those infants as transplant candidates. Recently, a series of 29 patients has been reported with 6.9% operative mortality and 86% actuarial survival at five years.[5] According to the tri-

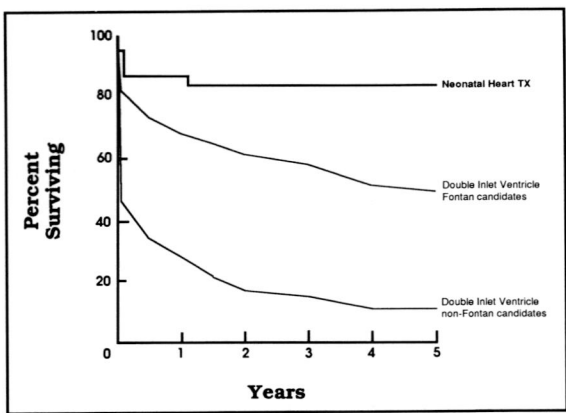

Fig. 2. Comparison between actuarial five-year survival after neonatal heart transplantation at Loma Linda Unviersity (n=52) and survival of patients with double inlet ventricle (n=191) from the combined experience of The Hospital for Sick Children and The Brompton Hospital in London, United Kingdom.[4] The 136 patients judged to be potentially suitable for a Fontan procedure at presentation had a better survival than the remaining 55, who were initially considered unsuitable for an atrio-pulmonary anastomosis.

partite classification of right ventricular morphology, seven of the 29 infants (24%) had an inlet-only right ventricle, and six of them had major right ventricular-coronary artery fistulas. Two patients in this subgroup died perioperatively and another two at subsequent operations for a total mortality of 47%; the remaining three patients were still awaiting definitive operations. Therefore, the subset of patients with pulmonary atresia, intact septum and inlet-only right ventricle should undergo early neonatal transplantation. Patients with both the inlet and the infundibular portion of the right ventricle should be transplanted in the presence of right ventricular-dependent coronary artery circulation.

Unbalanced atrioventricular septal defect

Repair of this lesion has been associated with poor results, even when the left ventricle is not extremely diminutive. In recent studies it has been appropriately included in the HLHS series. Thus it has been treated in the neonatal period with a Norwood procedure. Unfortunately, survival with the first stage has been less than 50%,[1] and transplant remains the only viable option.

Mitral valve disease

Congenital anomalies of the mitral valve requiring valve replacement in the first year of life have a one- and five-year survival rate of 52 and 43% respectively.[6] Furthermore, the operative survivors had an actuarial freedom from

repeat valve replacement of 45% at three years, and reoperative mortality was 11%. Severe mitral valve disease in early infancy would be better treated with heart transplantation.

Aortic stenosis

Critical valvular aortic stenosis in the first month of life is still connected with high mortality.[7] Isolated aortic stenosis may be treated with 0% hospital mortality, while association with other lesions increases the risk up to 47%. Hospital survivors with both isolated and complex aortic stenosis remain at significant risk, and the overall actuarial survival at 38 months is only 53%.

Aortic coarctation

Hypoplastic transverse arch and coarctation in neonates is not considered to be an indication for transplantation. Actuarial survival at five years is 72% in 66 newborns.[8] It is 87% in simple coarctation, 88% if a ventricular septal defect is present, 52% for complex coarctation. Neonatal complex coarctation might be an indication for transplantation.

Ebstein's anomaly

The symptomatic infant with Ebstein's anomaly has had a very poor prognosis in the past with an expected mortality greater than 50%, and it has been a clear indication for neonatal heart transplantation. A new surgical procedure has been recently developed to transform the lesion into tricuspid atresia, and orient the patient to a Fontan type of repair with satisfactory early results.[9]

PERSISTENT TRUNCUS ARTERIOSUS

The presence of truncal valve dysplasia resulting in significant postoperative aortic valve incompetence or stenosis has led to a poor operative outcome with conventional procedures, and these patients should undergo replacement therapy.

CORONARY ARTERY ANOMALIES

When these lesions are responsible for significant myocardial infarction and/or severe mitral regurgitation, they make up an obvious transplant category, fitting the criteria of end-stage myocardial disease.

EXPANDED INDICATIONS FOR NEONATAL HEART TRANSPLANTATION

There are numerous conditions for which neonatal heart transplantation is not presently considered acceptable treatment, since conventional palliative surgery seems to achieve reasonable results. But in many cases long-term results are not known and the advantages of reparative surgery are not defined.

FONTAN PROCEDURE CANDIDATES

A significant group is constituted by the so-called low risk Fontan candidates, which includes patients with tricuspid atresia and concordant ventriculoarterial connection. Operative mortality of the Fontan operation for tricuspid atresia has been reduced to 8%. After a mean follow-up of 5.5 years only another 3% are lost with 91% of the remaining patients being in excellent or good condition.[10] Unequivocal long-term results at 20 years or longer are not available, and it is not known whether the postoperative elevation of right atrial and systemic venous pressure will lead to a significant number of patients with protein-losing enteropathy, atrial dysrhythmias, and thromboembolic complications. Transplantation provides a backup therapy in the event a patient with

atriopulmonary connection is failing.

RIGHT VENTRICULAR OUTFLOW TRACT RECONSTRUCTION

RVOTR with a valved conduit can be achieved with low operative mortality and good intermediate term results.[11] Actuarial survival in 141 patients, aged two days to 35 years (mean 5.9 years), was 87% at five years, but freedom from conduit replacement was only 37% at five years. Considering the unimpressive difference in long-term performance between homograft and heterograft valved conduits, it is conceivable that these patients might be better served with transplantation as a primary definitive operation.

CONGENITAL HEART DISEASE WITHOUT TRANSPLANT INDICATION

In several congenital heart diseases transplantation is not considered to be indicated. Two main categories may be distinguished.

LOW RISK COMPLEX LESIONS

In some conditions the long-term results of a properly timed corrective operation appear to be superior to results achieved with cardiac transplantation. The neonatal Mustard operation for correction of simple transposition has a five-year survival of 91%.[12] The arterial repair in neonates with transposition and intact ventricular septum offers a five-year survival of 89%.[13] Babies with transposition and ventricular septal defect are better treated with the arterial switch operation, since survival at five years is 85%.[14] However, neonatal repair of tetralogy of Fallot[15] may not compare favorably with neonatal transplantation (Fig. 3), five-year survival being 74 and 84% respectively.

LOW RISK SIMPLE LESIONS

Atrial septal defects, single ventricular septal defects, atrioventricular septal defects with balanced ventricles, pulmonic stenosis, total anomalous pulmonary venous connection, and supracardiac aortic stenosis are not indications for transplantation.

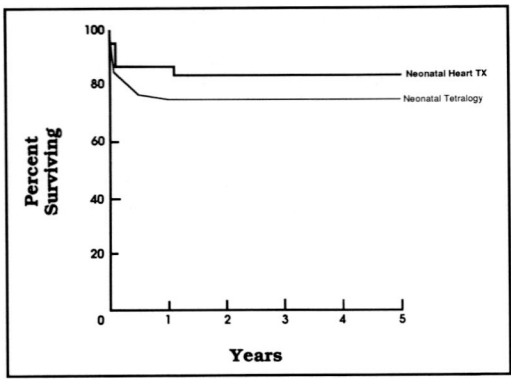

Fig. 3. Tetralogy of Fallot repaired in the neonatal period (n=27) at Children's Hospital of Boston.[15] Results are not different from neonatal heart transplantation at Loma Linda University (n=52).

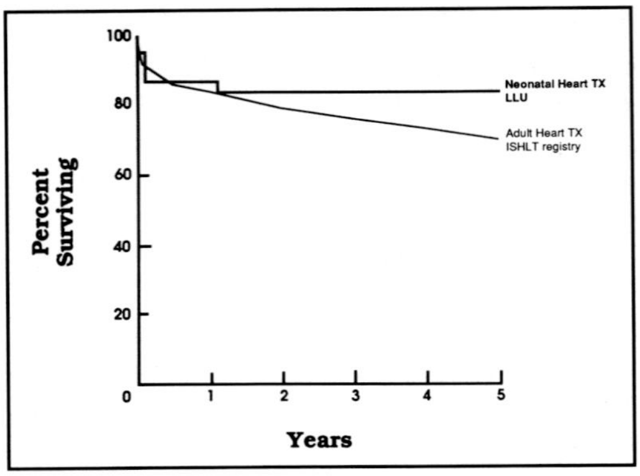

Fig. 4. Adult heart transplantation in United States in the years 1985-91. Result from the Registry of the "International Society for Heart and Lung Transplantation" (n=8332) are plotted with the transplant experience at Loma Linda University in newborns (n=52).

RESULTS OF NEONATAL HEART TRANSPLANTATION

The overall actuarial survival curve (Kaplan-Meier method) for newborns receiving heart transplantation is given in Figure 4. The actuarial survival is 84% at five years. These results compare favorably with the adult experience with cardiac transplantation. Adult data from the Registry of the International Society for Heart and Lung Transplantation during the same time period demonstrate a 70% survival at five years. It is encouraging that the neonatal survival curve becomes flat after the first year, whereas the adult population shows a constant attrition. These results suggest that a transplanted newborn, who survives the early months after the operation, should have excellent chances of long-term survival. If operative deaths and one late death due to hemorrhagic shock after circumcision are excluded in the Loma Linda experience, five-year survival is 95%. Neonatal heart transplantation is, therefore, effective therapy for complex incurable congenital heart anomalies and avoids the significant cumulative mortality, morbidity, and expense associated

with multiple palliative interventions. In the final analysis, there is no real substitute for normal cardiac anatomy and physiology. Loma Linda intermediate term results may allow expansion of indications for neonatal transplantation. (Table—see page 115) If the long-term results continue to be as favorable as the intermediate-term outcome, several additional congenital anomalies may be best managed with neonatal heart transplantation at the primary operation. Since transplantation is donor organ-dependent therapy, this entire discussion assumes a gradually evolving increase in available transplantable hearts in the infant age group. Maximizing donor resources will be the single most important issue as we implement the future of this incredible form of definitive therapy.

ACKNOWLEDGEMENT

We thank Dr. Michael P. Kaye who provided the data from the Registry of the International Society for Heart and Lung Transplantation.

Heart Disease Meeting Criteria for Orthotopic Transplantation in the Newborn

Treatment Class I

Conditions for which neonatal heart transplantation is indicated on the basis of a demonstrated advantage over conventional surgery in terms of longevity or relief of symptoms, or both.
1. Hypoplastic left heart syndrome
2. Univentricular atrioventricular connection with discordant ventriculoarterial connection
3. Pulmonary atresia with intact ventricular septum and inlet-only right ventricle and/or right ventricular-dependent coronary artery circulation (unless hypoplastic pulmonary arteries are associated)
4. Atrioventricular septal defects with unbalanced ventricles
5. Transposition with straddling atrioventricular valves
6. Critical valvular aortic stenosis
7. Mitral valve disease requiring valve replacement
8. Interrupted aortic arch type C, or any type associated with significant subaortic stenosis
9. Truncus arteriosus with truncal valve anomalies
10. Coronary artery anomalies with significant myocardial infarction and mitral regurgitation.
11. Cardiac tumors
12. Congenital cardiomyopathies

Treatment Class II

Conditions for which neonatal heart transplantation may be acceptable treatment, but for which its advantages over conventional surgery have not yet been defined.
1. Multiple ventricular septal defects ("Swiss cheese")
2. Univentricular atrioventricular connection with ventriculoarterial concordance
3. Atrioventricular septal defects with subaortic stenosis
4. Tetralogy of Fallot (requiring valved conduit insertion)
5. Pulmonary atresia, ventricular septal defect (requiring valved conduit insertion) without hypoplastic pulmonary arteries and/or major aortopulmonary collaterals
6. Transposition with ventricular septal defect and pulmonic stenosis
7. Double outlet right ventricle (requiring valved conduit insertion)
8. Atrioventricular discordance with ventriculoarterial concordance
9. Absent pulmonary valve syndrome
10. Ebstein's Anomaly (symptomatic in the newborn)
11. Subvalvular aortic stenosis
12. Truncus arteriosus

Treatment Class III

Conditions for which heart transplantation is not considered to be indicated.
1. Atrial septal defects
2. Ventricular septal defects
3. Atrioventricular septal defects with balanced ventricles
4. Tetralogy of Fallot (not requiring valved conduit insertion)
5. Pulmonary atresia, ventricular septal defect with hypoplastic pulmonary arteries and/or major aortopulmonary collaterals
6. Transposition with intact ventricular septum or isolated ventricular septal defect
7. Double outlet right ventricle (not requiring valved conduit insertion)
8. Anomalous venous connection
9. Interrupted aortic arch type A and B without subaortic stenosis
10. Aortic arch anomalies
11. Aortic coarctation (isolated or with ventricular septal defect)
12. Ductus arteriosus
13. Supravalvular aortic stenosis

References

1. Murdison KA, Baffa JM, Farrell PE, Chang AC et al. Hypoplastic left heart syndrome: Outcome after initial reconstruction and before modified Fontan procedure. Circulation 1990; 82 (suppl IV):IV-199-IV-207.

2. Farrell PE, Chang AC, Murdison KA, Baffa JM, Norwood WI. Outcome and assessment following modified Fontan repair for hypoplastic left heart syndrome. J Am Coll Cardiol 1990; 15:204A.

3. Franklin RCG, Sullivan ID, Anderson RH, Shinebourne EA, Deanfield JE. Is banding of the pulmonary trunk obsolete fr infants with tricuspid atresia and double inlet ventricle with a discordant ventriculoarterial connection? Role of aortic arch obstruction and subaortic stenosis. J Am Coll Cardiol 1990; 16:1455-64.

4. Franklin RCG, Spiegelhalter DJ, Rossi Filho RI, Macartney FJ et al. Double-inlet ventricle presenting in infancy. III: Outcome and potential for definitive repair. J Thorac Cardiovasc Surg 1991; 101:924-34.

5. Hawkins JA, Thorne JK, Boucek MM, Orsmond GS et al. Early and late results in pulmonary atresia and intact ventricular septum. J Thorac Cardiovasc Surg 1990; 100:492-7.

6. Kadoba K, Jonas RA, Mayer JE, Castaneda AR. Mitral valve replacement in the first year of life. J Thorac Cardiovasc Surg 1990; 100:762-8.

7. Karl TR, Sano S, Brawn WJ, Mee RBB. Critical aortic stenosis in the first month of life: Surgical results in 26 infants. Ann Thorac Surg 1990; 50:105-9.

8. Lacour-Gayet F, Bruniaux J, Serraf A, Chambran P et al. Hypoplastic transverse arch and coarctation in neonates. Surgical reconstruction of the aortic arch: A study of sixty-six patients. J Thorac Cardiovasc Surg 1990; 100:808-16.

9. Starnes VA, Pitlick PT, Bernstein D, Griffin ML et al. Ebstein's anomaly appearing in the neonate. J Thorac Cardiovasc Surg 1991; 101:1082-7.

10. Mair DD, Hagler KJ, Puga FJ, Schaff HV, Danielson GK. Fontan operation in 176 patients with tricuspid atresia: Results and a proposed new index for patient selection. Circulation 1990; 82 (suppl IV): IV-164-IV-169.

11. Sano S, Karl TR, Mee RBB. Extracardiac valved conduits in the pulmonary circuit. Ann Thorac Surg 1991; 52:285-90.

12. Alonso de Begona J, Kawauchi M, Fullerton D, Razzouk AJ, Gundry SR, Bailey LL. The Mustard procedure for correction of simple transposition of the great arteries before one month of age. J Thorac Cardiovasc Surg 1991, in press.

13. Planche CI, Serraf A, Lacour-Gayet F, Bruniaux J, Bouchart F, Comas J. Anatomic correction of transposition of the great arteries and intact ventricular septum in neonates; A study on 272 patients. In: D'Alessandro LC, ed. Heart Surgery 1991. Rome: CESI, 1990:247-55.

14. Serraf A, Bruniaux J, Lacour-Gayet F, Sidi D, Kachaner J, Bouchart F, Planche CI. Anatomic correction of transposition of the great arteries with ventricular septal defect; experience with 118 cases. J Thorac Cardiovasc Surg 1991; 102:140-7.

15. Di Donato RM, Jonas RA, Lang P, Rome JJ, Mayer JE, Castaneda AR. Neonatal repair of tetralogy of Fallot with and without pulmonary atresia. J Thorac Cardiovasc Surg 1991; 101:126-37.

CHAPTER 15

ARTIFICIAL ORGANS

Suzan A. McGary
Reed D. Quinn
William S. Pierce

INTRODUCTION

Less than 50 years have passed since the introduction of the heart-lung machine to the operating theater. In the short time since this landmark device was first utilized, the field of cardiac surgery has continued to develop and mature as technical innovations have allowed successful revascularization of ischemic myocardium, replacement and repair of diseased valves, repair or palliation of congenital defects, and when other treatments will not suffice, cardiac transplantation.

In 1989, more than 2,000 heart transplants were performed at 226 transplant centers worldwide.[1] An estimated 20% of potential transplant patients die of their heart disease before a suitable donor organ can be procured. There are also a significant number of patients who are not considered to be transplant candidates due to advanced age or concomitant medical problems such as diabetes or pulmonary hypertension. It is for these groups of patients that artificial organ development holds so much promise.

BRIDGE TO TRANSPLANTATION

PNEUMATIC VENTRICULAR ASSIST DEVICE (VAD)

The time between evaluation for a cardiac transplant and the actual procedure can range from mere days to many months. There are patients for whom the wait may be fatal. For many patients aggressive medical management with inotropic drugs and the intra-aortic balloon pump is helpful, but some require more.

Pneumatic VADs have been used successfully for up to 153 days as a means of support until a donor organ could be found.[2] These pumps are most commonly used for left ventricular support, but have also been placed for right ventricular and bilateral ventricular assistance.

Placement of the pneumatic VAD is a relatively uncomplicated procedure performed through a median sternotomy. An inflow cannula is placed in the atrium or ventricle to decompress the heart. Blood flows through a one-way tilting disc valve into the pump and is ejected through a second valve into a Dacron vascular graft which enters the proximal ascending aorta (or pulmonary artery for a right VAD) in an end-to-side fashion. (Fig.1) This method of insertion allows minimal disturbance of the myocardium and removal of the vascular suture lines of the mechanical device at the time of transplantation.[3] The pump itself is made of a flexible elastomer blood sac contained within a rigid plastic housing. The external drive unit introduces timed pulses of gas alternating with a slight vacuum between the blood sac and the housing to empty and

fill the sac. The VAD may be set manually at a desired rate or may be placed in an automatic mode in which rate is varied by the drive unit to maintain a given aortic pressure (or central venous pressure for a right VAD).[4]

The pump and drive unit are externally located with the cannulas passing transcutaneously. The drive unit is large and not considered portable, the patient is therefore tethered to this unit and may ambulate only in his room. (Fig. 2)

Despite the physical drawbacks, these devices have proven quite successful. A combined registry of all patients receiving mechanical assistance reports 23 patients receiving a left VAD and 33 patients receiving bilateral VADs in 1989. No right VADs were placed as a bridge to transplant during that year. Of those receiving left ventricular support, 12 (52.2%) were transplanted and 10 of those 12 (83.3%) were eventually discharged. In patients requiring bilateral ventricular assistance, 18 (54.6%) were

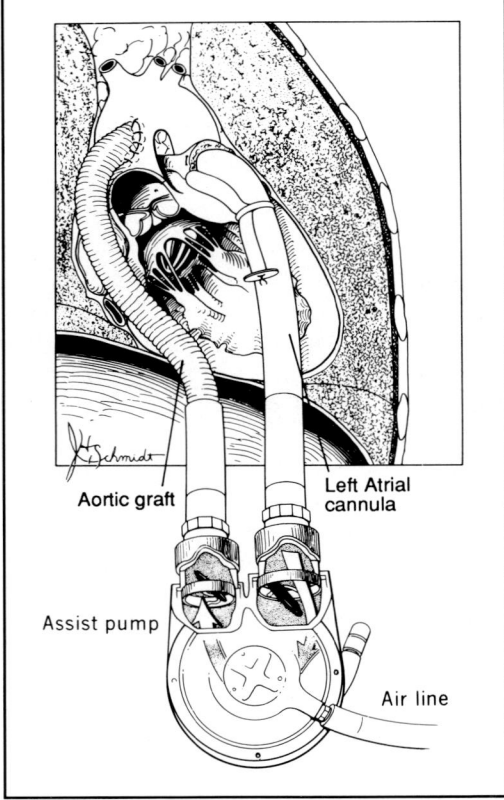

Aortic graft   Left Atrial cannula

Assist pump

Air line

Fig. 1. This sagittal view of the mediastinum demonstrates placement of a left VAD with atrial cannulation. The air line conducts a slight vacuum alternating with pulses of gas from the drive unit to facilitate filling and emptying of the assist pump. Blood flows into the left atrial cannula, past a one-way tilting disc valve into the blood sac and is pumped through a second valve into a Dacron vascular graft sewn end-to-side onto the aorta. This allows decompression of the left side of the heart.

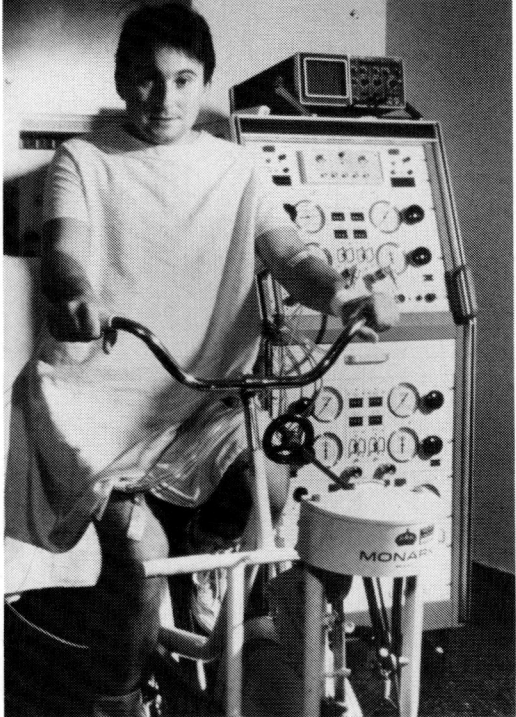

Fig. 2. The patient shown here has a pneumatic left VAD as a bridge to transplant. Notice that though he is able to perform low level exercise, the large drive unit behind him prevents him from venturing out of his room.

transplanted and of those 18, 12 (66.7%) were discharged from the hospital.[2]

PNEUMATIC TOTAL ARTIFICIAL HEART (TAH)

When VADs are used, the patient's own heart remains in place and can act as a back-up system should the VAD malfunction. For a few patients, for example those with a large ventricular aneurysm and thrombus, those with postmyocardial infarction ventricular septal defects, and those patients who have previously undergone cardiac transplantation and present with severe rejection, the heart itself is a threat and expeditious removal of the diseased heart can prevent neurologic injury from thromboemboli, pulmonary hypertension secondary to an acute VSD, or continuation of the rejection process which may lead to systemic complications.

The TAH offers temporary circulatory support in these situations while a donor heart is located. The current pneumatic model is placed in the chest much as an orthotopic transplant with anastomoses to the atria, pulmonary artery, and aorta. (Fig. 3) Drive lines cross the skin and connect the patient to a large bedside drive unit. The pneumatic TAH functions much like two VAD's placed together with intermittent pulses of gas from the drive unit alternating with a slight vacuum to facilitate emptying and filling of each blood sac. The right and left sides of the TAH function independently in regard to rate. Each side may be set manually to a desired rate or placed on automatic to allow variation of the rate. The right side is varied to maintain a given left atrial pressure and the left side a given aortic pressure.[4]

Patients who require this type of mechanical intervention are obviously poorer surgical risks than those who require only ventricular assistance. The combined registry report reveals that in 1989, 20 patients underwent placement of TAH as bridge to trans-

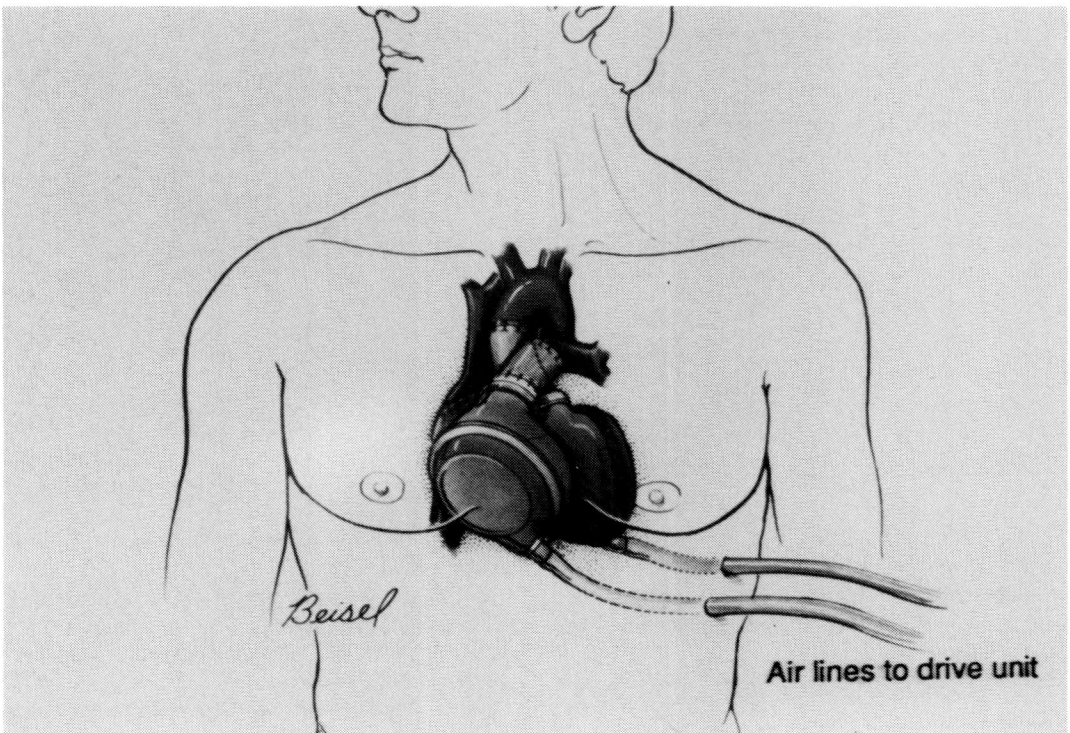

Fig. 3. The pneumatic TAH is placed in the chest in the same manner as an orthotopic heart transplant. The right side of the heart is anastomosed to the right atrial cuff and the pulmonary artery, the left side to the left atrial cuff and the proximal ascending aorta. Two air lines pass through the skin to an external drive unit which provides pulses of gas to the space between the blood sac and the rigid plastic housing to empty the pump and a slight vacuum to augment filling.

plant. Of these, 12 (60%) received a transplant. Of the 12 that were transplanted, only two (16.7%) were discharged from the hospital.[2]

ELECTRIC VENTRICULAR ASSIST DEVICE

Despite the relative success of the pneumatic pumps, they are cumbersome with large drive units and the transcutaneous cannulas place the already critically ill patient at risk for life-threatening infection. These units have therefore been refined and modified with much work directed toward development of a more compact device with a less bulky power source. The result has been the electric VAD.

Designed in the fashion of the pneumatic pump, the device is inserted in the same way with the exception that the pump is placed into a preperitoneal pocket through a separate abdominal incision. In current models, such as those in designed by Novacor Medical Corporation and the newly approved Thermedics device, a cable is passed from the pump transcutaneously to an electric power source which supplies power to an implanted miniature prime mover—either a rotary solenoid or a brushless direct current motor.[4] The electric drive unit is much more compact and is portable, allowing patient mobility.

In 1989, 17 patients received an electric VAD as a bridge to transplant. Of those, eight (47.1%) underwent transplantation. Of the eight patients receiving transplants, six (75%) were discharged from the hospital.[2]

These devices have undergone extensive animal trials; similar units at our institution placed in young Holstein calves have functioned well for four and five months. The electronics have proven to be reliable. Animal deaths are most commonly due to calcification and rupture of the blood sacs. Blood sac calcification has been a common problem in the calf model but is not anticipated to cause difficulty in the clinical setting.[5]

PERMANENT DEVICES

Due to the limited number of acceptable donor organs available, age limits and restrictions concerning the health of the recipient (excluding the heart disease itself) consider-

able effort is utilized to best place the available organs into younger, healthier individuals. In the years to come, those patients not considered suitable for transplantation may have the option of permanent assist device placement or placement of a permanent TAH6.

Current models of VADs, including the newly approved electric devices made by Thermedics and Novacor, all have some component passing through the skin. This prevents their practical utilization in these critically ill patients for more than a few weeks or months. Long-term use of these devices is fraught with complications of infection along the transcutaneous cables or cannulas. In order to perfect a permanent device, transcutaneous passage of any portion of the device has to be eliminated. The solu-

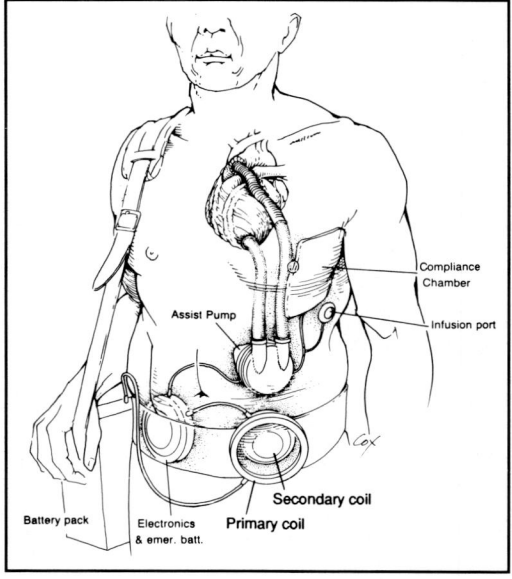

Fig. 4. This drawing depicts an electric VAD in place on the left side of the heart. The small external battery pack allows nearly unlimited mobility for the patient. This battery pack can provide up to 6 hours of uninterrupted power before being recharged on a house current. An internal battery which can power the unit for up to 30 minutes provides a back up system in the event of external power loss. In addition, these patients retain their own hearts which, in case of mechanical or electrical failure, can provide at least some circulatory support until the device can be repaired or replaced.

tion is a fully implantable VAD or TAH powered by a small, portable electric power pack. Power will be delivered to the unit using the principle of inductive coupling. A primary coil located on the skin and held in place with a belt will transmit power transcutaneously to a secondary coil located subcutaneously. The power pack will be equipped with batteries which provide up to six hours of energy to the VAD or TAH before being recharged on a house current. An internal battery system will provide emergency power for 30 minutes in the event of loss of or separation from the external power source. The external power source will be small, about the size of a briefcase, allowing

the patient full mobility for the six hours of energy provided by the batteries.[7] (Figs. 4 and 5)

Most patients (approximately 70%) in this population will require only an assist device, their own hearts remaining in place. The remaining 30% are those whose hearts are a threat to their lives and continued well being and who would benefit from cardiectomy and circulatory support from a TAH. The indications for cardiectomy would be, for example, a patient with a large ventricular aneurysm with associated thrombus and poor left and right ventricular function.

Patients receiving the implantable devices would require frequent monitoring, especially those with TAHs since they no longer have their native heart to act as a backup system as do the VAD patients. The initial clinical life of these pumps is expected to be one to two years with ongoing improvements and modifications increasing the useful life span to five or more years before the units need to be replaced. Experience with the implanted electric VAD will come sooner than that for the TAH and lessons learned from the VAD will be applied to the TAH to decrease the incidence of malfunction in these rather vulnerable patients.

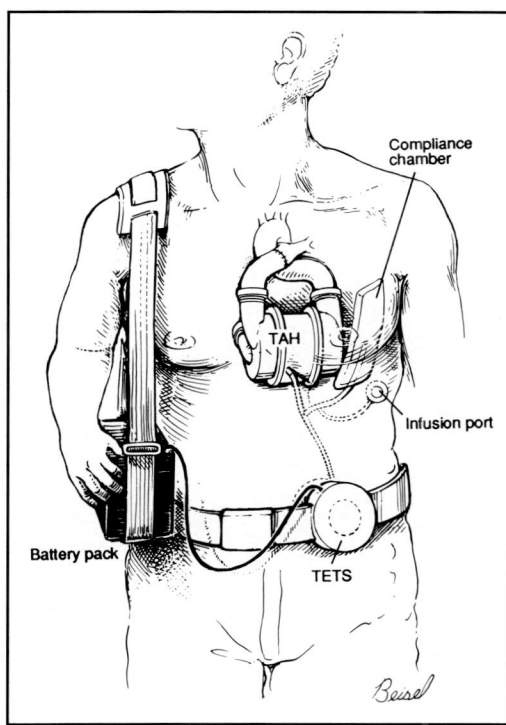

Fig. 5. The totally implantable electric motor artificial heart is placed in the chest much like an orthotopic heart transplant with anastomoses to the pulmonary artery, aorta, and right and left atria. Power is provided by an external battery pack and transmitted transcutaneously via inductive coupling. A primary coil is held on the skin with a belt and a secondary coil is placed subcutaneously. Internal batteries can provide up to 30 minutes of back up power in the event of separation from or loss of the external power source.

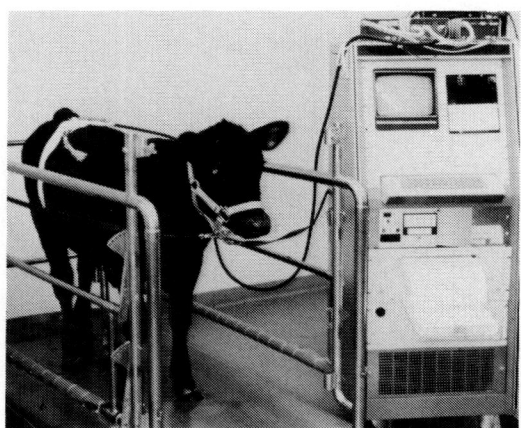

Fig. 6. This calf lived more than 200 days after cardiectomy and placement of an electric TAH. Her postoperative course was without complication—she was alert and active and grew normally. The transcutaneous drive line can be seen exiting from her right side and extending to the drive unit on the left.

Animal studies are underway and totally implanted devices (VAD and TAH) will be placed in young Holstein calves in the coming year. (Fig. 6)

SUMMARY

The progression of successful surgical intervention in cardiac disease is proceeding rapidly. Current techniques of cardiopulmonary bypass, vascular bypass grafting, valve repair and replacement, and cardiac transplantation have helped thousands lead more normal lives. The technology of the future, including electric motor VADs and TAHs promises to extend that normalcy to others whose illness is not readily addressed by today's methods. This includes patients with both acute and chronic disease for whom current therapies are inadequate. Like pacemakers and intra-aortic balloon pumps, as production and implantation techniques of mechanical assist devices progress, they will become more widely available—stock items in operating rooms across the country. Prices for the devices will decrease as the ability to produce the components in significant quantities is realized.

These continuing advancements will allow us to offer a quality life to patients whose cardiac status today means long term debility or premature death. (Fig. 7)

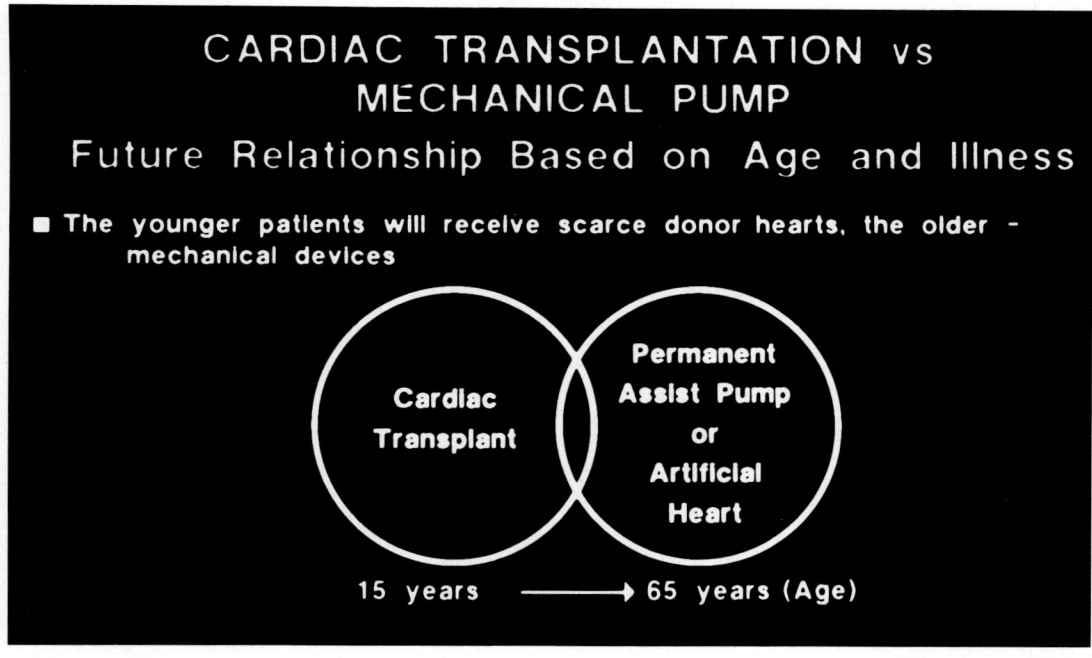

Fig. 7. With the clinical use of implantable VADs and TAHs cardiac transplantation in the future can be reserved for the young, otherwise healthy individual while the older patient or the patient with contraindications to transplantation can be treated with mechanical assistance. An estimated 70% of those receiving implantable devices will require only ventricular assistance. The remaining 30% will undergo placement of a TAH after cardiectomy. These devices will give the transplant surgeon options previously not realized for patients whose current prognosis is grim.

REFERENCES

1. Kriett JM, Kaye MP. The registry of the international society for heart transplantation: Seventh official report-1990. J Heart Transplant 1990; 9(4):323-30.

2. Miller CA, Pae WE, Pierce WS. Combined registry for the clinical use of mechanical ventricular assist pumps and the total artificial heart in conjunction with heart transplantation: Fourth official report-989. J of Heart Transplant 1990; 9(5):454-58.

3. Pierce WS. Horizons in Assisted Circulation. Assisted Circulation 1989; 3:614-15.

4. Jurmann MJ, Pae WE, Wisman CB, Miller CA, Pierce WS. Mechanical Circulatory Assistance for End-Stage Myocardial Failure. Progress in Cardiology 2/2 1989; 241-58.

5. Pierce WS, Myers JL, Donachy JH, Rosenberg G, Landis DL, Prophet GA, Snyder AJ. Approaches to the Artificial Heart. Surgery 1981; 90(2):137-48.

6. Pierce WS. The Use of Mechanical Circulatory Support in Advanced Congestive Heart Failure. Congestive Heart Failure 1982; 329-35.

7. Pierce WS, Pae WE, Myers JL, Waldhausen JA. Cardiac Surgery: A Glimpse Into the Future. J Am Coll Archiol 1989; 14(2):265-75.

CHAPTER 16

CARDIAC XENOTRANSPLANTATION

Hermann Reichenspurner

Bruno Reichart

INTRODUCTION

The need for use of xenotransplantation has become more and more evident because of the lack of suitable human donor organs. This scarcity of donors is compounded further by the fact that transplantation of the heart may be necessary as an emergency procedure. There is a clearly defined need for heart transplantation in neonates and infants. Severe cardiac defects, such as hypoplastic left heart syndrome, have a poor prognosis after conventional cardiac surgery, but organ procurement for neonates remains a major problem. The use of anencephalic infant donors raises additional ethical and legal restrictions.[1] The only biological option to an allogeneic graft is therefore a xenogeneic donor heart.

Suppression of the immune response is particularly important in the xenogeneic model due to the occurrence of early hyperacute and severe cellular rejection. Cyclosporine (CyA), in addition to its well known use in allogeneic transplantation, has also been described as prolonging graft survival in the xenogeneic model.[2,3,4] Before CyA became available, conventional immunosuppresive drugs like azathioprine, corticosteroids or antilymphocyte globulin (ALG) were used to avoid graft rejection. Dubernard and Donawick described ALG as being able to prolong renal, cardiac and skin xenograft survival in an experimental model.[5,6]

The effect of CyA on xenograft survival has been controversial. Homan et al were able to extend the survival of hamster hearts, transplanted heterotopically into rats, only by administering toxic dosages of CyA.[2] In the hamster-to-rat xenograft model, suppression of mainly humorally mediated rejection episodes was achieved by CyA only in combination with splenectomy of the recipient.[7] In contradistinction, Bailey et al have described a significant increase in survival of lamb hearts in newborn goats with the use of CyA.[8] Michler et al reported on a 12-fold increase of graft survival after cardiac xenotransplantation in primates using parenteral CyA and corticosteroids.[9] Experiments carried out in the fox/dog model have shown an improvement in heart xenograft survival time using immunosuppression with CyA in combination with methylprednisolone.[3] In several other experimental studies, the positive effect of CyA has not been confirmed and it has been suggested that the success of CyA is dependent on the various animal species being used.[10]

As another form of immunosuppressive therapy, total lymphoid irradiation (TLI) was reported to be effective after cross-species transplantation, particularly when combined with ALG.[11] The combination of CyA and TLI led to a prolongation of heart xenograft survival in the hamster/rat model;[12] graft survival was greater than 100 days in most of these animals. In our own laboratory experience, when the combination of CyA and TLI was used in primates, the occurrence of rejections was decreased significantly, but severe treatment-related complicatons were the major cause of death in the experimental animals.[13]

The major aim of this research protocol was to optimize immunosuppressive therapy after xenogeneic transplantation. The present study shows the influence of different immunosuppressive drug combinations with CyA on xenograft survival, as well as on occurrence and number of hyperacute and acute cellular rejection episodes. A particular point of interest was the combination with a new immunosuppressive agent, 15-deoxyspergualin.

In addition, the possibility of clinical xenotransplantation is discussed extensively and preconditons and contraindications are mentioned.

EXPERIMENTAL ANIMALS, MATERIAL AND METHODS

Donor and recipient animals

In order to avoid early hyperacute rejection, as it occurs in discordant xenograft models, a concordant xenograft model was chosen by using Vervet monkeys as donors and Chacma baboons as recipients. According to evolution studies, the genetic disparity of these two animals is comparable to the model chimpanzee-homo sapiens.[14]

Vervet monkeys *(Cercopithecus aethiops)*

weighing two to six kg served as donors in our xenograft model. Chacma baboons *(Papio ursinus)* weighing 10 to 15 kg were used as recipients. The donor and recipient animals were matched and compatible within the AB blood group system.

All animals received care according to the: "Ethical considerations in medical research, revised edition: 1987" set out by the South African Medical Research Council, Parow, 1989.

Anesthesia and surgical technique

After premedication with ketamine (5 mg/kg b.w.), morphine (0.25 mg/kg b.w.), pancuronium bromide (0.2 mg/kg b.w.) and atropine (0.5 mg), anesthesia was maintained with a combination of halothane (1%)\ oxygen 4 L/min and N_2O 6 L/min as inhalation.

The operative technique of heterotopic heart transplantation in the neck was used according to the technique of Mann et al.[15] After a median sternotomy, the pericardium was opened longitudinally in the donor animal. After ligation of both venae cavae and crossclamping of the aorta, the heart was perfused with cold cardioplegic solution. All pulmonary veins were ligated and the heart was explanted.

In the recipient animal, the carotid artery and internal jugular vein were prepared in the right neck. The donor's aorta was the anastomosed end-to-side with the carotid artery of the recipient and the donor's pulmonary artery with the right internal jugular vein. Thus, the heart graft was placed heterotopically in the right neck of the recipient. (Fig. 1)

Immunosuppressive protocol

Based on immunosuppressive regimens, the following groups were studied (Table 1):

Group I (n=8) served as a control group with no immunosuppression given.

Group II (n=5) received CyA in a dosage of 20 to 40 mg/kg/day administered intramuscularly, according to a whole blood trough level aimed at between 400 and 600 ng/ml. CyA was combined with azathioprine (2.5

Table 1. Immunosuppressive protocol in the different groups after heterotopic cardiac xenotransplantation.

Groups	Immunosuppressive Protocol
I	control, no immunosuppression
II	CyA 20-40 mg/kg/d + aza 2.5 mg/kg/d + mp 0.3 mg/kg/d
III	CyA + aza + mp + RATG 9-15 mg IgG/kg/d, p.o.d. 0-4
IV	CyA + aza + mp + 15-DS 3 mg/kg/d, p.o.d. 0-4, 2mg/kg/d, p.o.d. 5-9
V	CyA + mp + 15-DS 4 mg/kg/d, p.o.d. 0-9

Cya = cyclosporine A, asa = azathioprine, RATG = rabbit antithymocyte globulin, 15-DS = 15-deoxyspergualin

mg/kg/day) and methylprednisolone (0.3 mg/kg/day tapered down to 0.2 mg/kg/day over 3 weeks).

Group III (n=6): In addition to the drug regimen of group II, rabbit antithymocyte globulin (RATG, Fresenius, Frankfurt, Germany) in a dosage of 9-15 mg IgG/kg/day was given for postoperative days 0-4.

Group IV (n=7): In this group, the triple-drug regimen of group II consisting of cyclosporine (CyA), azathioprine and methylprednisolone, was combined with 15-deoxyspergualin (15-DS, 3 mg/kg/day administered intravenously for postoperative days 0-4 and 2 mg/kg/day for postoperative days 5-9). Due to severe treatment related side effects which were

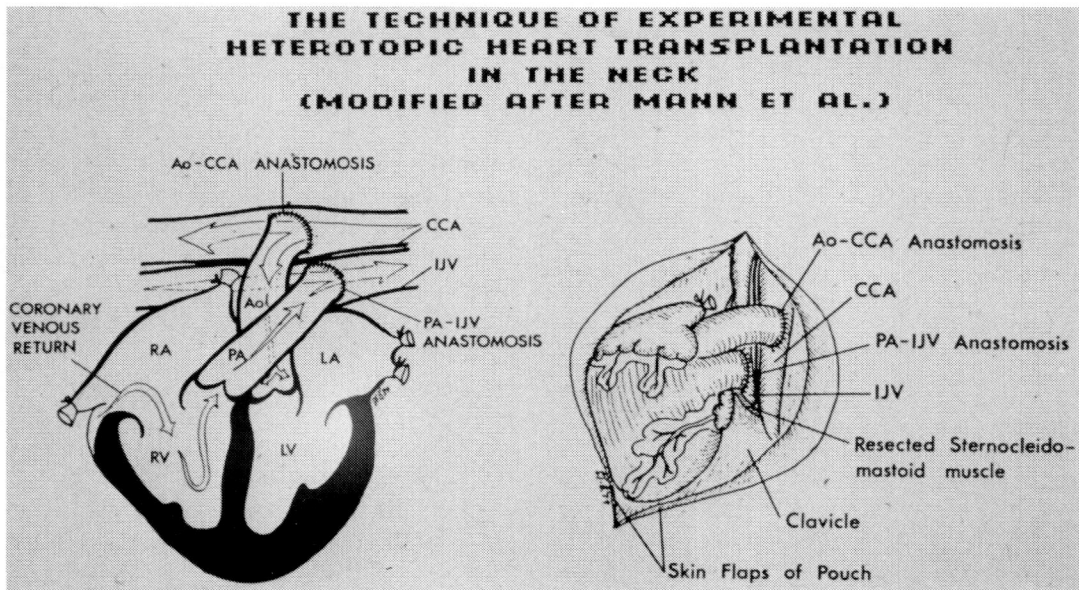

Fig. 1. Operative technique of heterotopic heart transplantation in the neck according to the technique of Mann[5] (CCA = common carotid artery, IJV = internal jugular vein, Ao = ascending aorta, PA = pulmonary artery).

observed in this group, the immunosuppression was modified as follows:

In group V (n=5), 15-DS (4 mg/kg/day administered intravenously for postoperative days 0-9), was combined with CyA and methylprednisolone only, and azathioprine was omitted. In addition, the infusion time of 15-DS was prolonged to 3 hours of continuous intravenous infusion.

Acute rejection episodes were treated with 500 mg methylprednisolone intravenously for 3 to 5 consecutive days in groups II-V.

POSTOPERATIVE MONITORING

Every day after transplantation, the graft function was checked and the heart was palpated by one specific person. In addition, the animals underwent a full clinical examination.

Three times weekly, blood samples were taken for routine hematological, biochemical and cytoimmunological monitoring.

At weekly intervals, transmyocardial biopsies were performed. For this procedure, the animals were briefly anesthetized (ketamine 5 mg/kg, halothane 1%, N_2O, O_2) and a small skin incision was made above the transplanted heart. The transmyocardial biopsy was then performed using a trucut biopsy needle and a full thickness biopsy was taken through the left ventricular wall.

The biopsies were evaluated histologically and rejection episodes were divided into three groups according to the histopathology:

1. *Acute cellular rejection.* Perivascular and interstitial mononuclear cell infiltration combined with interstitial edema and/or presence of myocyte necrosis. (Fig. 2)

2. *Hyperacute rejection.* Extensive interstitial edema and hemorrhage combined with myocyte necrosis and presence of neutrophil granulocytes. Mononuclear cell infiltration is missing. (Figs. 3,4)

3. *Mixed rejection.* The biopsy findings in this group show features of both the acute cellular and hyperacute type of rejection. (Fig. 5)

STATISTICS

Statistical significance was calculated in accordance with the Log rank analysis or the Student t test.

RESULTS

GRAFT SURVIVAL

The experiments were terminated whenever the grafts stopped functioning or when the animal died of any other complication. The survival rates for the different groups are shown in Figure 6 and Table 2.

The control group I with no immunosuppression had a mean graft survival of 10.3 ± 5.4 days.

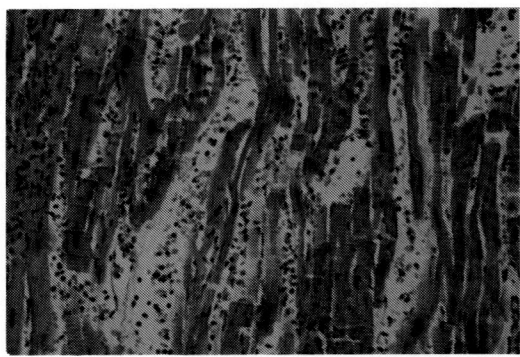

Fig. 2. Acute cellular rejection after cardiac xenotransplantation: A similar picture occurred after allotransplantation: Mononuclear cell infiltration occurs perivascularly and in the interstitium, in combination with myocyte necrosis and interstitial edema.

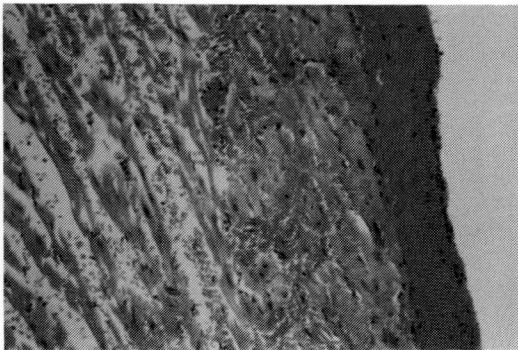

Fig. 3. Hyperacute rejection after xenogeneic transplantation: interstitial hemorrhage, interstitial edema and myocyte necrosis is seen without any mononuclear cell infiltrate.

Treatment with CyA, azathioprine and methylprednisolone (group II) led to a mean graft survival of 19.0 ± 21.8 days and showed no significant difference to the untreated control group.

The addition of RATG to the immuno-suppressive protocol (group III) led to a significantly higher survival time of 43.3±18.5 days (p<0.005 vs. control). The most successful experimental animal lived for 77 days after transplantation.

The combination of the basic drug regimen with 15-DS (group IV) also increased the graft survival rate to 20.1±11.5 days (p<0.05 vs. control). The omission of azathioprine in this drug regimen consisting now of CyA, methylprednisolone and 15-DS (from postoperative day 0-9) improved graft survival even more to 35.6±14.2 days on average (p<0.01 vs control group, Table 2).

Causes of experiment termination and treatment-related side effects

The causes of experiment termination are graphically illustrated in Figure 7.

In groups I and II, cellular and hyper-acute graft rejection were the dominant causes of graft failure in 89% and 80% of the animals respectively. When RATG was added (group III), acute rejection terminated the graft function in 50% of the cases, while infections, diarrhea and other complications such as thrombosis of the graft anastomoses or renal failure were the cause of death in the remaining 50%.

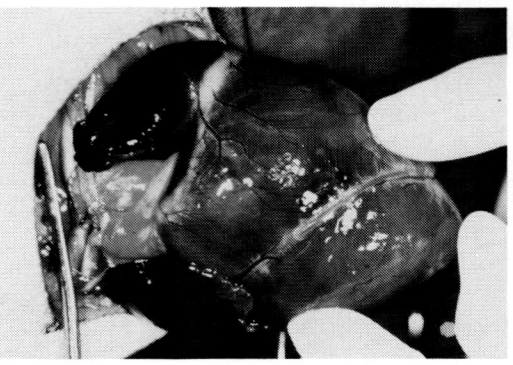

Fig. 4. Macroscopic picture of hyperacute rejection; note the swelling of the heart and the hemorrhage on the surface.

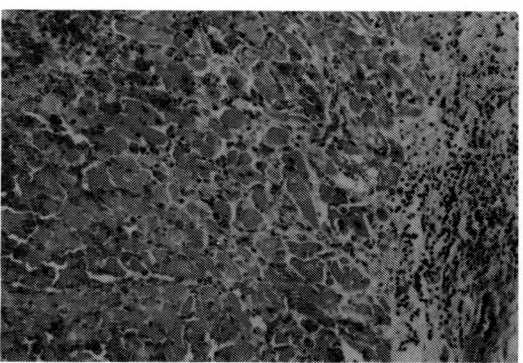

Fig. 5. Mixed type of acute rejection after xenogeneic transplantation. In addition to the above demonstrated features of hyperacute rejection, typical signs of cellular rejections are seen such as mononuclear interstitial cell infiltrations.

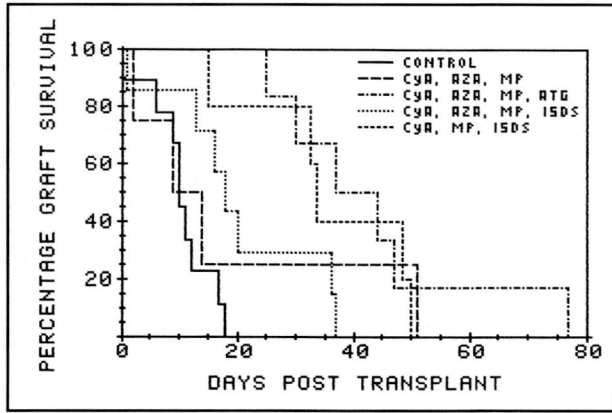

Fig. 6. Xenograft survival rates for the different treatment groups. The best graft survival rate was achieved with a combination of CyA, azathioprine, methyl-prednisolone and RATG (group III). The termination of graft survival within the first 2 days postoperatively corresponded always to the occurrence of hyperacute rejection.

Table 2. Graft survival rate (GSR) in days after cardiac xenotransplantation within the different groups I-V.

Groups	I	II	III	IV	V
GSR	10.3	19.0	43.3***	20.1*	35.6**
(days)	±5.4	±21.8	±18.5	±11.5	±14.2

***p<0.005   **p<0.01   *p<0.05 vs. control

The combination of the triple-drug regimen with 15-DS led to a high incidence of lethal complications, such as infections and diarrhea in 57% of the animals. The remaining 43% of the experiments were terminated due to graft rejection.

Omission of azathioprine (group V) results in fewer treatment related side effects; 80% of the animals were sacrificed due to graft rejection and only 20% died of infections.

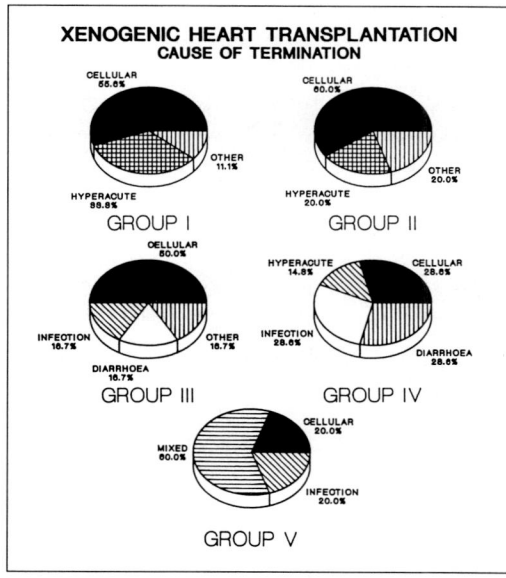

Fig. 7. Causes of experiment termination shown graphically in pie diagrams. Rejections (hyperacute, cellular or mixed) were the dominant causes in groups I and II, while infections and gastrointestinal complications occurred mainly in groups III and IV. In group V, less lethal treatment related side effects were seen.

NUMBER OF ACUTE REJECTIONS

The number of rejection episodes per animal was calculated for each group and is listed in Table 3.

In group II, an average of 1.5 rejection episodes per animal was observed. In group III, the group with the longest survival rate, 2.5 acute rejections per animal were nevertheless observed and had to be treated.

The results were significantly different in the 15-DS treated groups. In group IV only 0.5 graft rejection episodes occurred per animal (p<0.05 group IV vs. groups II and III). In group V also only 0.8 rejections per animal were observed, although survival and observation periods are similar to group III (p< 0.05 vs group III).

Table 3. Number of acute rejections per animal in each treatment group. In group IV only 0.5 and in group V only 0.8 rejections per animal were observed. This number differed significantly from the results obtained in group III.

Group	I	II	III	IV	V
AR (n)	1.0	1.5	2.5	0.6*	0.8*

p<0.05 vs group III

AR = acute rejection episode

HISTOPATHOLOGY OF ACUTE REJECTION

In the control group I, hyperacute rejections were seen in 33.3% of the animals, mixed rejections in 55.6% and cellular rejections in 11.1% (Fig. 8). This means that in nearly 90% of all biopsies, there were features of acute rejection in the biopsy findings.

In the treated groups II, III and IV, hyperacute rejections occurred less frequently. In group II, only 14.3% of the rejections were hyperacute and 21.4% of mixed type, 21.4% of rejections were of the cellular type and 41.9% of the biopsies turned out to be normal. In group III, hyperacute rejection occurred in only 10.8% of the animals, cellular rejections in 35.1% and mixed rejections in 40.5% Despite having the longest survival rate, only 18.5% of the biopsies in this group showed normal myocardium with no evidence of rejection.

In both 15-DS treated groups IV and V, the majority of all biopsy samples were normal and showed no signs of rejection. In group IV, 74.7% of the biopsies showed normal myocardium. Only 4.5% hyperacute rejections occurred; 18.2% of the rejections were of cellular and 4.5% of mixed origin. In group V, 61.5% of the biopsies were normal, while 19.2% of the biopsy samples showed rejections of the cellular type and 19.2% rejections of the mixed type. (Fig. 8)

CONCLUSION

The combination of CyA with azathioprine and methylprednisolone did not show a significant increase in xenograft survival rate in this model. These findings confirm those by Sadeghi et al who used a similar experimental model in primates.[16]

The triple-drug regimen with the addition of rabbit antithymocyte globulin (RATG), however, led to a highly significant prolongation of experimental duration resulting in the longest graft survival time achieved. A recent publication by Michler et al confirms the success of this drug regimen including RATG after xenotransplantation in primates.[17]

The use of 15-DS instead of RATG and omission of azathioprine resulted in a significantly improved survival time in group V.

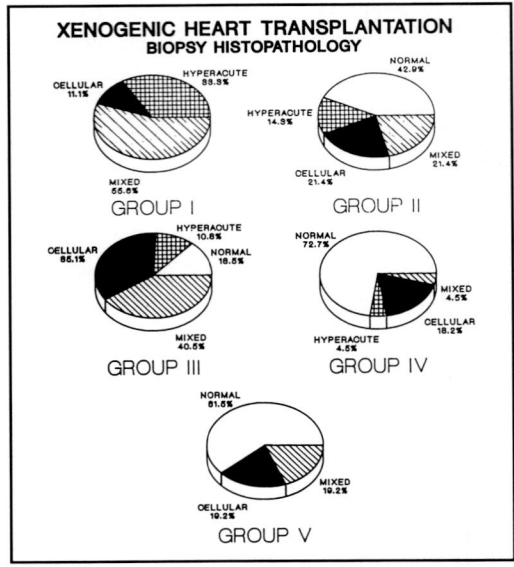

Fig. 8. Histopathology of the myocardial biopsies. Most of the biopsy findings in groups I, II and III showed evidence of rejection; in groups IV and V, 72.7 and 61.5% of the results were normal with no sign of acute rejection.

Graft survival in this group was not significantly different from results achieved in the group with RATG (group III).

Thomas et al have also described 15-DS as being a potent immunosuppressive drug for xenotransplantation.[18] Particularly in combination with RATG, optimal results were achieved after mouse-to-rat skin transplantation.

In group III (33%) and particularly in group IV (53%), infections and severe treatment related side effects, such as diarrhea and emaciation, were the main reasons for termination of the experiments. This high rate of complications occurring in group IV led to a modification of the 15-DS protocol in group V. Omission of azathioprine and a combination of 15-DS with CyA and methylprednisolone only, resulted in a decrease of treatment related side effects and thus provided a significant prolongation of animal survival time.

The most prominent finding in groups IV and V was the fact that 15-DS was able to reduce the number of hyperacute and acute cellular rejection episodes significantly.

In the 15-DS treated group V, no hyperacute rejection episode occurred, and 61.5% of all histology results were negative with regard to acute rejection. Also in the 15-DS treated group IV, over 70% of the biopsy results were normal with no evidence of rejection features.

Thus 15-DS treatment led not only to a decreased number of acute rejection episodes, but also to a lowered incidence of severe hyperacute rejections.

This is particularly important, because it has been shown in earlier studies after xenogeneic transplantation that the acute cellular type of rejection can be treated with additional antirejection therapy in contrast to vascular or hyperacute rejection episodes.[3]

These demonstrated experimental results achieved in our laboratory as well as those reported by the mentioned authors, are very stimulating.

In the concordant model, where hyperacute rejection occurs less often, the immune response seems to be under better control using specific immunosuppressive drug combinations.

Using the concordant species system, clinical xenotransplantation should be possible in the near future, at least as a bridging procedure in emergency situations.

Before clinical application, the following preconditions must be considered in accordance with Bailey and coworkers.[4]

Pretransplant immunological tests should include at least six individual animals: A mixed lymphocyte culture is necessary in which the responsiveness of recipient lymphocytes to the cells of the potential donor is examined in order to select the most suitable donor animal. In addition, the usual direct lymphocytotoxic crossmatch should be performed. The presence of maternal antibodies must, however, be considered and excluded before final evaluation.

ABO-compatibility is essential; it is condition *sine qua non*. Since primates such as baboons or Vervet monkeys do not have the blood group O, neonates and infants with blood group O cannot be considered for xenotransplantation.

Postoperatively, every blood transfusion administered to the transplant recipient should be tested for lymphocytotoxic antibodies against the donor animal and for CMV-seronegativity. Only irradiated packed cells,

after four repeated washings, should be used.

Finally, nonhuman primates are known to harbor a substantial population of viral species that could cause serious disease or death, especially in the immunosuppressed transplant recipient.[19] Prior to their utilization as organ donors in the clinical setting, therefore, these animals must be screened for viruses such as the Herpes simplex type, cytomegalovirus, the simian immunodeficiency retrovirus and other human immunodeficiency virus species related to the retroviral strains.[19]

In the discordant system, which ultimately seems to be the desirable xenotransplant model, the presence of preformed natural antibody remains a formidable obstacle. Suppressing the immune response after discordant xenotransplantation is at present not possible due to the occurrence of severe early hyperacute rejection. Transplant research in this field should aim, in the final analysis, at modulation of antigen recognition rather than influencing the immune response.

REFERENCES

1. Harrison ME. Organ procurement for children: The anencephalic fetus as donor. Lancet ii:1983,1986.
2. Homan WP, Williams KA, Fabre JW et al. Prolongation of cardiac xenograft survival in rats receiving cyclosporin A. Transplantation 1981; 31:164.
3. Reichenspurner H, Ertel W, Reichart B, Peters D et al. Xenogeneic and allogeneic canine heart transplantation: A model for cytologic and immunologic monitoring of rejection mechanisms. J Heart Transplant 1986; 5: 471.
4. Bailey LL, Nehlsen-Cannarella SL, Concepcion W, Jolley WB. Baboon-to-human cardiac xenotransplantation in a neonate. JAMA 1985; 254:3321.
5. Dubernard JM, Bonneau M, Bonel J et al. Renal and skin xenografts from baboons to macaques: Effect of antilymphocyte globulins. Transpl Proc 1971; 3:545.
6. Donawick WJ, Shaffer CF, Dodd DC et al. Cardiac and skin heterograft rejection: Suppression with antilymphocyte serum. Transp Proc 1971; 3:551.
7. Valdivia LA, Monden M, Gotoh M et al. An important role of the spleen in rejection of hamster-to-rat xenografts. Transpl Proc 1988; 20:329.
8. Bailey LL, Jang J, Johnson W, Jolley WB. Orthotopic cardiac xenografting in the newborn goat. J Thorac Cardiovasc Surg 1985; 89:242.
9. Michler RE, McManus RP, Smith CR et al. Prolongation of primate cardiac xenograft survival with cyclosporine. Transplantation 1987; 44:632.
10. Sugimoto K, Shelby J, Corry RJ. The effect of cyclosporine on cardiac xenograft survival. Transplantation 1984; 39:218.

11. Hardy MA, Oluwole S, Fawwaz R et al. Selective lymphoid irridation: Prolongation of cardiac xenografts and allografts in presensitized rats. Transplantation 1982; 33:237.

12. Knechtle SJ, Halperin EC, Saad T, Bollinger RR. Prolonged heart xenograft survival using combined total lymphoid irridation and cyclosporine. J Heart Transplant 1986; 5:254.

13. Cooper DKC, Huamn PA, Reichart B. Prolongation of cardiac Xenograft (vervet monkey to baboon) function by a combination of total lymphoid irradiation and immunosuppressive drug therapy. Transpl Proc 1987; 19:4441.

14. Human PA, Reichenspurner H. Heart and heart lung transplantation - orthotopic and heterotopic techniques. In: Reichart B, Jamieson SW, eds. Verlag, Percha, FRG: RS Schulz, 1990:267-277.

15. Mann FC, Priestly JT, Markowitz J, Yater WM. Transplantation of the mammalian heart. Arch Surg 1983; 26:219.

16. Sadeghi AM, Robbins RC, Smith CR et al. Cardiac xenotransplantation in primates. J Thorac Cardiovasc Surg 1987; 98:809.

17. Michler RE, Margoe CC, Socha WW et al. Simian-type blood group antigens in nonhuman primate cardiac xenotransplantation. Transpl Proc 1987; 19:4456.

18. Thomas RT, DeMasi RJ, Hugh D et al. Comparative immunosuppression for xenografting. In: Hardy MA, ed. Excerpta Medica Amsterdam-New York-Oxford 1989:55-66.

19. Van der Riet F, Human PA, Cooper DKC et al. Virological implications of the use of primates in xenotransplantation. Transplant Proc 1987; 19:4068.

CHAPTER 17

NEW TRENDS IN LUNG PRESERVATION: A COLLECTIVE REVIEW

Richard J. Novick

Alan H. Menkis

F. Neil McKenzie

INTRODUCTION

Because of its delicate alveolar-capillary membrane network, the lung exhibits a marked sensitivity to ischemia. This factor, coupled with our still incomplete understanding of the pathogenic mechanisms involved in pulmonary ischemia-reperfusion injury, has caused the long-term preservation of lung grafts to lag behind the preservation of other organs for transplantation.

In the seven years since the last major review of this topic,[1] successful lung transplantation has become a clinical reality and considerable strides have been made in the experimental laboratory in understanding the optimal conditions for the procurement, storage and reperfusion of lung grafts. With the growing experience in bilateral sequential lung transplantation,[2] ischemic times of over six hours are now commonplace in clinical practice. Nevertheless, pulmonary dysfunction following lung and heart-lung transplantation is still distressingly frequent.[3] The next few years will witness the further clinical application of knowledge gained in experimental lung transplantation in an effort to improve the function of lung grafts following long-term preservation.

This review highlights the strategies that have been employed recently in the experimental laboratory in order to minimize ischemia-reperfusion injury after lung transplantation. The first section will review new experimental models of lung preservation that have been proposed since 1985. Subsequent sections will examine in detail research directed at optimizing lung graft procurement and storage, as well as interventions during the reperfusion phase to prevent post-ischemic lung damage.

EXPERIMENTAL MODELS OF LUNG PRESERVATION

The past few years have witnessed the publication of several new experimental models of lung transplantation, which appear to offer significant advances over traditional methods in determining the adequacy of lung allograft preservation. Although experimental models of heart-double lung[4] or heart-unilateral lung[5,6] transplantation continue to be reported, most investigators have focused on the transplantation of isolated lung allografts, in order to eliminate the confounding variable of cardiac preservation. Furthermore, the duration of lung allograft preservation has been lengthened in most recent reports, and storage intervals of at least 12 hours (and as long as 30 hours) are now regarded as standard in the lung preservation literature.

In 1988 the University of Toronto group reported a new model of canine left lung transplantation in which the right and left pulmonary arteries were encircled with inflatable cuffs which were connected to subcutaneous reservoirs.[7] Sequential inflation of each cuff produced complete pulmonary artery occlusion and enabled comparison of the function of the transplanted lung to the normal contralateral lung immediately postoperatively and several days later. This model permitted the study of both acute preservation-related lung injury and the delayed manifestations of ischemia-reperfusion lung damage, and has been subsequently employed in the comparison of intracellular and extracellular pulmonary flush solutions in 12-hour lung preservation.[8]

In 1990, Bonser and associates reported an en bloc double lung transplant model in dogs, with reperfusion after 12 hours of hypothermic lung storage.[9] The function of the transplanted lungs was assessed by repeated measurement of lung mechanics, hemodynamics, gas exchange and pulmonary shunt fraction. Whereas traditionally PO_2 has been believed to be the most sensitive discriminator of appropriate lung preservation,[1,10] this experiment showed that promi-

nent pulmonary mechanical changes occur after prolonged hypothermic ischemia, and that these alterations are also sensitive indices of allograft function. The main disadvantage of this model is the need for cardiopulmonary bypass, which complicates the experimental design and has potentially damaging effects on lung function.

Over the past few years, there has been a recrudescence of isolated perfused working lung models for the assessment of lung preservation. The major advantage of these models is the ability to control lung volume as well as perfusate flow and composition more accurately than in intact animal preparations, and to measure lung edema formation continuously as the gain in lung weight.[11] Their principal disadvantage is the tendency of the isolated perfused lung to develop pulmonary hypertension and edema spontaneously, following a shorter preservation interval than in intact animal preparatons.[11]

Recently, LoCicero and associates have developed a prototypic model of isolated, perfused canine lungs which provides sensitive on-line measurements of their aerodynamic, gas exchange and hemodynamic characteristics, without the confounding variables of chest wall and pleural fluid dynamics or post-thoracotomy pain.[12,13] This model has subsequently been employed for the comparison of crystalloid and colloid (University of Wisconsin) solutions[14] and for the investigation of the role of bronchial artery flushing in prolonged lung preservation.[15,16]

Over the past three years, the University of Toronto and Washington University groups have employed a simple ex vivo rabbit lung preparation in which the left lung is perfused with autologous venous blood for 10 minutes after a prolonged ischemic interval, with measurement of gas exchange, airway pressure and pulmonary vascular resistance. This model has been used to study the effects of ischemic time and storage temperature,[17] the effect of verapamil,[18] and to compare low-potassium dextran solution to Euro-Collins solution in prolonged lung preservation.[19] Recently, the model was modified to prolong the reperfusion interval from 10 to 60 minutes using a paracorporeal circulation through an anesthetized support rabbit.[20] The chief advantage of the ex vivo rabbit lung model lies in its relative simplicity, low cost and reliability.[17] It is an excellent screening method to examine the myriad factors influencing lung allograft preservation, and helps to direct the study of specific aspects of lung preservation in intact animals prior to their potential clinical application.

Because of the large variety of experimental models that have been used to assess the efficacy of pulmonary preservation, published results from different centers have at times been contradictory. This underlines the necessity of standardizing not only the types of models employed in lung preservation research, but also the criteria by which lung preservation is analyzed and reported in the literature.

ORGAN PROCUREMENT

The conduct of the organ procurement procedure in experimental and clinical lung transplantation is one of the most important variables affecting the functional status of the allograft postoperatively. Clinically, four methods of lung preservation have been employed: donor core-cooling on cardiopulmonary bypass, single flush perfusion of the lungs followed by static cold storage, topical cooling of the lungs followed by static cold storage, topical cooling of the lungs after absorption atelectasis,[21] and normothermic autoperfusion of the heart-lung block.[22] The third and fourth methods were used during the early clinical experience with lung and heart-lung transplantation, respectively, and are now mainly of historical interest. Although practised in only a few centers, donor core cooling on bypass has been employed in over 50% of the world's experience in heart-lung transplantation.[23-25] Conversely, single flush perfusion of the lungs is by far the most widely used technique in clinical lung preservation today.

Donor Core Cooling

Cardiopulmonary bypass and deep donor hypothermia without flush perfusion of the lungs has provided reliable lung preservation for four hours in experimental heart-lung transplantation in calves[26] and for six hours in dogs.[5,27] Inadequate lung preservation has

resulted after 12 hours of cold storage with this technique, unless an oxygen free radical scavenger was added during harvest, preservation and reperfusion.[28]

The literature comparing experimental lung preservation with donor core cooling to single flush perfusion of the lungs is conflicting. In calves, heart-lung grafts preserved for four hours following donor core cooling exhibited less extravascular lung water and improved lung biopsy scores as compared to heart-lung grafts in which lung preservation was provided by pulmonary artery flushing with Euro-Collins solution with prostaglandin E_1 pretreatment.[26] In dogs undergoing heterotopic heart-left lung transplants, preservation was similar in the donor core cooling and pulmonary artery flushing groups, except for a significant reduction in pulmonary vascular resistance following donor core cooling.[5,27]

Conversely, in primates, heart-lung grafts preserved with modified Euro-Collins pulmonary flush with high dose prostaglandin E_1 exhibited superior oxygen transfer after six hours of storage as compared to heart-lung grafts procured by donor core cooling.[29] Similarly, in a canine single lung transplant model with ligation of the contralateral bronchus and pulmonary artery, pulmonary artery flushing with cold modified blood and prostacyclin was clearly superior to donor core cooling after six hours of hypothermic storage.[30]

In the only comparative (but non-randomized) clinical study to date, allograft function following heart-lung or single lung preservation with simple hypothermic flush was as good as or better than that following extracorporeal circulation.[31] Because of the lack of clear evidence in the experimental transplant literature that donor core cooling is superior, and the excellent results, lower cost and simplicity associated with single flush perfusion of the lungs, the latter has become the most widely practiced technique in lung transplantation in recent years.[32]

Single Flush Perfusion Technique

Composition of the pulmonary flush solution. Historically, a wide variety of perfusates have been utilized in experimental lung preservation.[1] Prior to 1986, none of these provided sufficient pulmonary protection to enable routine distant donor procurement. In that year the Stanford group reported the successful six-hour preservation of primate heart-lung allografts using a hypothermic pulmonary artery flush with 60 ml/kg of modified Euro-Collins solution, followed by static hypothermic storage.[33] The realization that 60 ml/kg of pulmonary perfusate administered over several minutes at a low pressure resulted in a more uniform cooling of the lungs than the lower flush volumes previously employed was a major advance in experimental lung preservation.[34] In the following year, Baldwin and associates reported the successful application of this technique to clinical heart-lung transplantation,[35] adding impetus to the evolving clinical experience with long distance heart-lung and lung allograft procurement. A further experimental study using six-hour canine lung preservation[10] confirmed the superiority of Euro-Collins pulmonary artery flush to topical cooling alone. Since that time, modified Euro-Collins solution has become the standard pulmonary flush solution in most centers practicing clinical lung and heart-lung transplantation.

Synchronous with the Stanford experience with a hypothermic crystalloid pulmonary flush solution, the Papworth group reported the use of an extracellular blood-based solution containing prostacyclin for distant heart-lung procurement.[36,37] A follow-up report in 1990 confirmed that this technique provides satisfactory lung preservation for up to four hours in most patients.[38] To date only one comparison of modified blood versus Euro-Collins pulmonary artery flush has been conducted in a canine lung transplant model.[39] PO_2s during the reperfusion phase after six hours of cold preservation were not different between groups, but lungs flushed with modified cold blood demonstrated significantly lower compliance and accumulated significantly more water during reperfusion. The authors concluded that modified Euro-Collins solution with added prostacyclin provides good lung preservation for six hours, and may be superior to pulmonary artery flushing with cold modified blood containing the same dose of prostacyclin.[39]

Low-potassium dextran solution. Further efforts to extend the interval of lung allograft preservation have been undertaken in recent years by investigating alternatives to Euro-Collins as a pulmonary flush solution. Work from Japan in the mid-1980s indicated that a modified crystalloid extracellular fluid may be superior to the intracellularly-based Euro-Collins solution as a pulmonary flush prior to prolonged lung allograft preservation.[40,41] The University of Toronto group, employing the dog single lung transplant model described above, found that an extracellular low-potassium dextran flush solution provided significantly better immediate function of the 12-hour preserved lung than did Euro-Collins solution; at three days postoperatively, however, oxygen transfer was not significantly different between groups.[8] The superiority of low-potassium dextran solution over Euro-Collins was confirmed in the isolated rabbit lung model after 18 hours of cold storage by the same group of investigators.[19] However, both of these studies were criticized because of the omission of donor prostaglandin therapy prior to flushing of the allograft. Euro-Collins solution is known to cause pulmonary vasoconstriction,[42] and it is conceivable that the beneficial effects of low-potassium dextran solution may have been due to less pulmonary vasoconstriction during lung harvest rather than to a specific effect of the low-potassium dextran solution during cold storage. In a subsequent study of 18-hour canine lung preservation in which allografts were pretreated with prostaglandin E_1 and then flushed with either low-potassium dextran or Euro-Collins solution, no significant difference in transplanted lung gas exchange or hemodynamic function was found immediately after reperfusion or at three days.[43] Modified Euro-Collins solution in conjunction with prostaglandin therapy has therefore continued to be used by most centers engaged in clinical lung transplantation.

University of Wisconsin solution. The recent introduction of Belzer-University of Wisconsin solution has significantly prolonged the preservation of liver,[44] kidney[45] and pancreatic[46] grafts, and altered the conduct of clinical liver transplantation by allowing truly long-term allograft preservation.[47] Experience with University of Wisconsin solution in experimental lung preservation is increasing, and the preponderance of evidence to date supports its beneficial role.

LoCicero and associates first contrasted the preservation provided by University of Wisconsin solution versus Euro-Collins solution in an isolated perfused working lung model after 130 minutes of cold storage.[12] Euro-Collins - preserved lungs exhibited worse shunt fractions and capillary leak, but aerodynamic measurements of lung resistance were significantly higher in the University of Wisconsin group.[12,14] In isolated preserved rat lungs, Semik and associates[48] found a slight advantage to University of Wisconsin solution over Euro-Collins solution after 8 and 24 hours of hypothermic preservation. Finally, Kawahara and associates found significantly worse airway pressure, lung compliance and pulmonary vascular resistance following 24 hours of cold storage of isolated canine lungs flushed with Euro-Collins versus University of Wisconsin solution, although post-reperfusion PO_2s were not significantly different and both groups of lungs exhibited massive weight gain.[49]

Experience with Belzer-University of Wisconsin solution for in vivo animal lung transplant models is limited. Naka and associates[50,51] noted superior function of canine heterotopic heart-left lung grafts following 24 hours of hypothermic storage after flushing with University of Wisconsin solution as opposed to modified Collins solution. In the University of Wisconsin group, there was no difference between pre- and post-transplant arterial PO_2 values, although pulmonary vascular resistance and lung water increased significantly.[50,51] In a canine single lung transplant model with ligation of the contralateral pulmonary artery and bronchus, 24-hour lung preservation with University of Wisconsin solution in conjunction with prostaglandin E_1 produced excellent gas exchange and only a modest increase in pulmonary vascular resistance.[52] This data was similar to that previously reported by the same investigators following six hours of pulmonary preservation with Euro-Collins solution.[10] The

Mayo Clinic and other groups have since begun to employ University of Wisconsin solution in clinical lung transplantation, with acceptable early results.

Despite the favorable initial experience with University of Wisconsin solution in experimental lung preservation, several important questions concerning its use remain unanswered. Standard University of Wisconsin solution is an intracellular solution containing a high potassium concentration (120 mmol/L), akin to that in Euro-Collins solution (115 mmol/L). Studies have revealed that a modified University of Wisconsin solution with a low potassium (9 mmol/L) and a high sodium content is effective in the preservation of dog liver, kidney and pancreas grafts.[53] This modified solution has recently been investigated in the isolated rabbit lung model by the University of Toronto group. After 30 hours of storage at 10°C, grafts flushed with low potassium University of Wisconsin solution exhibited superior gas exchange and less edema during reperfusion than lungs treated with standard (high potassium) University of Wisconsin or Euro-Collins solutions.[54] The authors concluded that in the absence of a pulmonary vasodilator, a high potassium concentration in the hypothermic pulmonary flush solution may cause pulmonary vasoconstriction and a non-uniform flush, yielding suboptimal pulmonary preservation notwithstanding other components of the preservation solution.

Future studies will need to investigate the effects of the various components of University of Wisconsin solution on lung preservation. Recent experiments have indicated that lactobionate, raffinose and glutathione are indispensable for liver preservation, whereas all other components appear to be dispensable.[55] Furthermore, the efficacy of University of Wisconsin solution in long-term cardiac preservation has been shown by Wicomb to be clearly related to its shelf-life.[56] Wicomb has postulated that one of the problems associated with shelf-stored University of Wisconsin solution is the conversion of reduced glutathione, an important neutralizer of cytotoxic oxygen free radicals and lipid peroxides, to oxidized glutathione.

Astier and Paul have demonstrated that after four months of storage of University of Wisconsin solution, reduced glutathione is completely converted to the oxidized form,[57] and Wolkowicz and Caulfield have shown that 12-month-old University of Wisconsin solution causes extensive degradation of cardiac collagen.[58] None of the studies employing University of Wisconsin solution for experimental lung preservation has specified the shelf-life of the flush solution or altered any of its components except for its potassium and sodium concentrations. The future of University of Wisconsin solution in lung preservation may be promising, but more work is required before it may supplant Euro-Collins as the standard flush solution in clinical lung transplantation.

Donor pretreatment prior to lung flushing. Historically, a myriad of substances have been administered to lung donors in an effort to improve the function of lung allografts after transplantation. The most commonly investigated drugs have included prostaglandins, corticosteroids, and calcium blockers. In many studies one or more oxygen free radical scavengers have been infused in a "shot-gun" fashion during lung harvest, preservation and reperfusion. Since the main role of these agents is to mitigate oxygen free radical damage post-transplantation, their use is reviewed in the section on reperfusion below.

Prostaglandins. Donor treatment with prostaglandin E_1 is a common clinical practice in North America, whereas in Europe prostacyclin is used routinely in lung allograft procurement. A recent paper has reviewed comprehensively the role of both of these prostaglandins in experimental and clinical lung transplantation.[59] Prostaglandins have a wide variety of actions that are of theoretical advantage in lung transplantation. Not only are they potent pulmonary vasodilators, but they favorably modulate white cell and platelet function by attenuating leukocyte sequestration in damaged tissues, inhibiting platelet aggregation, and preventing lysosomal enzyme release and superoxide anion production by neutrophils.[59] Furthermore, prostaglandins mitigate the vascular permeability that is induced by vasoactive inflammatory mediators

and have a pronounced cytoprotective effect.[59]

The preponderance of evidence supports the beneficial role of prostacyclin treatment of the donor in experimental lung and heart-lung transplantation, with only one study in the literature failing to demonstrate improved preservation in prostacyclin-treated lung allografts.[60] The role of prostaglandin E_1 in extended lung allograft preservation remains controversial, with studies in the past year from two centers showing no benefit.[59,61] A recent experiment by the University of Toronto group, however, demonstrated that prostaglandin E_1 treatment of the donor prior to flushing and 18 hours of cold storage improved the suboptimal lung preservation provided by Euro-Collins solution.[43] The dose of prostaglandin E_1 employed in this study was approximately 2.5 µg/kg/min, several times the dose used in the other two experiments. The issue as to whether donor prostaglandin E_1 therapy is truly beneficial awaits additional experimental studies, or, perhaps, a prospective randomized clinical trial.

Corticosteroids. Increasing evidence points to the importance of activated neutrophils in the etiology of acute lung injury.[62] Corticosteroids favorably alter granulocyte function by reducing lysosomal enzyme release and superoxide anion production by neutrophils.[63] In addition, corticosteroids inhibit complement-induced neutrophil aggregation[64] and block granulocyte arachidonic acid metabolism possibly by inhibiting phospholipase A2 activity.[63]

All three studies on corticosteroids in the lung preservation literature support their beneficial role in the mitigation of pulmonary ischemic injury. Hall and associates noted improved compliance, histology and edema in isolated rabbit lungs pretreated with pharmacologic doses of methylprednisolone and subjected to 12 hours of cold storage.[65] In isolated reperfused canine lobes, Matsumura and associates demonstrated a marked reduction in pulmonary capillary permeability with methylprednisolone treatment prior to 3 hours of warm ischemia and upon reperfusion.[63] Furthermore, a recent experiment by Hooper and associates in an in situ canine model showed improved oxygen transfer and pulmonary vascular resistance and less pulmonary edema when methylprednisolone was administered prior to one hour of normothermic lung ischemia.[66] Based on these results, donor treatment with pharmacologic doses of methylprednisolone should be investigated further in a large animal lung transplant model, and may merit consideration in clinical lung transplantation.

Calcium Blockers. Aside from activated neutrophils, calcium ion appears to be an important mediator of ischemia-reperfusion injury in many organs.[67] Intracellular calcium increases during hypothermia as well as during periods of ischemic injury.[68] An augmented intracellular calcium concentration may activate phospholipases and other enzymes, with the resultant synthesis of vasoactive arachidonic acid metabolites.[68] Calcium channel blockers have proved beneficial in models of kidney, heart and brain ischemia,[18] and these agents have recently been investigated in lung preservation.

Hachida and Morton have demonstrated that incorporating verapamil into the pulmonary flush solution improved oxygen transfer and pulmonary hemodynamics following normothermic lung ischemia[69] and six-hour hypothermic lung preservation[70] in dogs. Verapamil did not prevent impaired lung allograft function after 12 hours of cold storage, however.[71] Recent work by the University of Toronto group has revealed that in isolated rabbit lungs preserved by cold saline immersion alone, verapamil administered prior to lung extraction was more beneficial than verapamil infused only at reperfusion.[18] After flushing with low-potassium dextran solution, gas exchange after 30 hours of 10°C storage was equivalent with or without verapamil.[18] The authors concluded that prolonged ischemic times were required to demonstrate any benefit to verapamil pretreatment in lungs flushed with a hypothermic extracellular solution.[18] Further research is currently being undertaken with other calcium channel blockers such as diltiazem,[72] nifedipine[72] and nicardipine (Dr. Michael Kaye, personal communication, 1991) in an effort to ameliorate further pulmonary damage function following prolonged ischemia and reperfusion.

The potential role of bronchial artery perfusion in donor lung procurement. Most studies on lung preservation have ignored the role of the bronchial circulation despite the fact that this circulation supplies important nutrients to the intrapulmonary airways, bronchovascular bundles and walls of the pulmonary arteries and veins.[15,73] LoCicero and associates, using an isolated perfused working lung model, demonstrated a lower intrapulmonary shunt fraction, better compliance and less pulmonary granulocyte sequestration in lungs flushed with Ringer's lactate solution by both the bronchial and pulmonary circulations than by either route alone.[15] A follow-up report from the same group compared the 17-hour preservation of isolated canine lungs that were flushed with either Ringer's lactate or University of Wisconsin solution via both the pulmonary and bronchial circulations.[16] The University of Wisconsin group exhibited a lower shunt, lower airway resistance and decreased pulmonary granulocyte sequestration. In both experiments, the bronchial circulation was accessed by clamping the ascending aorta, great vessels and distal thoracic aorta, and by infusing the perfusate into this 15 cm closed aortic segment incorporating the origins of the bronchial vessels. In view of these encouraging preliminary results, further experiments in intact animal lung transplant models are warranted to ascertain whether dual pulmonary and bronchial artery flushing may confer any benefit in conditions mimicking clinical lung transplantation.

LUNG ALLOGRAFT STORAGE

OPTIMAL TEMPERATURE AND STORAGE MEDIUM

It has long been known that storage temperature is an important factor in lung preservation.[1] Normothermic lungs resist ischemia for only 30 minutes,[74] and deflated canine lungs maintained at normothermic ischemia for over an hour do not support life.[75] Hypothermia prolongs successful lung preservation,[76,77] but profound hypothermia might be deleterious to cellular membrane transport mechanisms and calcium hemostasis.[68] At the time of the last major review on lung preservation, no systematic investigation of the effects of storage temperature on lung allograft function had yet been reported.[1]

Over the past few years, this work has been undertaken in the isolated rabbit lung model by the University of Toronto group. Wang and associates studied six groups of lung preserved by topical saline immersion alone at temperatures ranging from 4°C to 38°C for one to 30 hours.[17] Moderate hypothermia improved ischemic tolerance, as measured by oxygen uptake, gas exchange and pulmonary artery pressure during reperfusion. Preservation at 10°C was significantly better than at 4°C and 15°C; oxygen transfer after 24 hours of ischemia at 10°C compared favorably to that following 12 hours of ischemia at 4°C or 15°C.[17] A follow-up study investigated the optimal temperature for pulmonary flushing with low-potassium dextran and Euro-Collins solutions.[78] Results were significantly better in the low-potassium dextran than in the Euro-Collins groups. After 18 hours of storage, the PO_2 was significantly higher in the low-potassium dextran lungs preserved at 10°C than at 4°C.[78] Euro-Collins' preserved lungs at 4°C exhibited a higher pulmonary artery pressure on reperfusion but a similarly poor PO_2 to lungs flushed and stored in 10°C Euro-Collins solution. The authors concluded that 10°C appears to be the optimal temperature for the long-term preservation of rabbit lungs. Further work in other animal models is required before a definitive statement can be made concerning the optimal temperature for graft storage in clinical lung transplantation.

The traditional technique of lung storage after procurement has been immersion in cold saline or iced-slush. One of the main problems with this approach has been inhomogeneous cooling of the graft due to buoyancy of the lung.[79] In addition, temperatures of portions of the graft completely submerged in an iced-slush bath could readily decrease below freezing, with resultant cryogenic lung injury.[80] Shimokawa and associates reported a method of topical lung cooling by ambient compressed air in conjunction with dry ice in a canine model of left lung transplantation.[79] Unfortunately, a relatively short ischemic time and no control group were employed in this ex-

periment. A more comprehensive investigation of the role of cold air storage has recently been published.[81] Canine lungs were excised without flushing and stored in either an iced-slush cooler at 0 to 4°C or in a commercially available container that keeps the lung cool with air at a constant, controllable temperature. After eight hours, lung grafts stored in cold air at 4°C, 8°C, and 12°C exhibited significantly better oxygen transfer and less extravascular lung water than grafts immersed in an iced-slush bath.[81] Further investigations are indicated in lung grafts undergoing pulmonary artery flushing prior to storage before this method could be recommended for routine clinical use.

Lung Inflation versus Deflation during Storage

Research in the early 1970s indicated that the duration of tolerable lung ischemia may be prolonged if the lungs remained ventilated or inflated during the ischemic interval.[75] Nevertheless, the group that pioneered successful clinical lung transplantation made a point in their early experience of keeping the allograft deflated with a bronchial blocker during procurement.[21,82] Immersion of the collapsed lung in cold saline provided satisfactory lung preservation in the majority of patients for up to four hours.[21]

In recent years the pendulum has swung definitively to the side of lung inflation during hypothermic storage. Locke and associates have shown that preservation following pulmonary artery flushing with Euro-Collins solution and lung inflation is superior to the preservation provided by topical cooling alone following absorption atelectasis of the lung.[10] A recent study in a canine single lung transplant model found improved 30-hour lung preservation in allografts that were hyperventilated prior to flushing and again immediately prior to tracheal clamping.[83] Mean PO_2s during reperfusion in these allografts were greater than 500 mm Hg on 100% oxygen whether or not prostaglandin E_1 was administered prior to lung harvest.

The issue as to the concentration of oxygen which should be administered to lung grafts immediately prior to storage remains an open question. Koyama and associates subjected isolated canine lobes to room temperature ischemia for six hours while ventilating them with either 100% oxygen, room air or 100% nitrogen.[84] By four hours of reperfusion, lobes ventilated with 100% oxygen or room air had incurred massive weight gain; lobes ventilated with 100% nitrogen were significantly less edematous. Pretreatment of lobes ventilated with room air or 100% oxygen with an oxygen free radical scavenger resulted in mitigation of the acute lung injury. The authors postulated that pulmonary ischemia-reperfusion damage was related to oxygen metabolites produced during ischemic ventilation, and that this damage could be minimized by ventilating with 100% nitrogen during the ischemic period.

Contradictory to this report is the recent finding by the Washington University group of improved 24-hour hypothermic preservation of isolated rabbit lungs inflated with 100% oxygen as opposed to room air.[20] Lungs stored in 100% nitrogen deteriorated even more rapidly than those inflated with room air upon reperfusion, and precipitously developed pulmonary edema. The authors reasoned that intraalveolar oxygen may be used by the lung during cold storage, and that the availability of oxygen during ischemia may be important for optimal lung preservation. Their results are weakened somewhat by the failure to measure oxygen free radical formation during reperfusion. Further work is clearly indicated to determine whether lung allografts should be inflated with oxygen-free or oxygen-rich gases immediately prior to a prolonged storage interval.

REPERFUSION

Despite optimal techniques of harvest and storage, the lungs are exquisitely sensitive to reperfusion injury after prolonged preservation. Reperfusion lung damage is likely a complex interplay of various pathogenic mechanisms, including leukocyte[85,86] and platelet[4] activation, oxygen-free radical formation,[85,86] the complement cascade, and the generation of inflammatory mediators and arachidonic acid metabolites.[87]

There is incontrovertible evidence in the literature that cytotoxic oxygen-free radicals are produced following both warm[88,89] and cold[85] lung ischemia. The pathobiology of oxygen-free radicals and the lung's endogenous defenses against cytotoxic oxygen metabolites are reviewed in detail elsewhere.[90-92] Oxygen-free radicals may originate from several sources during ischemia, including activated neutrophils, dissociation of the intramitochondrial electron transport chain and the xanthine oxidase reaction.[85,86,93] During ischemia the xanthine dehydrogenase enzyme is converted to xanthine oxidase, which catalyzes the formation of oxygen-free radicals when adenosine metabolism is accelerated during reperfusion.[86] The superoxide anion that is produced may act directly to damage cellular components or may give rise to singlet oxygen which is also cytotoxic.[90,91] The superoxide anion may also take part in the reduction of hydrogen peroxide to the very reactive hydroxyl radical by the Haber-Weiss reaction, with iron as the major catalyst.[90] The hydroxyl radical then initiates a chain reaction of extensive protein degeneration and lipid peroxidation in pulmonary endothelial cell membranes, leading to their increased permeability and the ultimate occurrence of pulmonary edema.[85] Independent verification of the direct toxic effect of oxygen-free radical generation on pulmonary endothelial cell function has already been demonstrated in isolated perfused rat lungs.[94]

Since the previous review on lung preservation in 1985, a number of strategies have been developed to combat reperfusion lung injury. These include the use of leukocyte filters to minimize the deleterious effects of activated neutrophils, xanthine oxidase inhibition with allopurinol, iron chelation with deferoxamine to inhibit the Haber-Weiss reaction, the infusion of oxygen-free radical scavengers, and the use of recently developed platelet-activating factor antagonists.

LEUKOCYTE DEPLETION

In an effort to prevent pulmonary leukostasis and neutrophil-mediated oxygen free radical release, since 1985 the Johns Hopkins group has investigated the role of reperfusing lung grafts with leukocyte-depleted blood. Early studies in isolated rabbit lungs showed improved 24-hour lung preservation when the initial reperfusate did not contain white cells.[95,96] Leukocyte depletion was achieved by passing the reperfusate through a commercially-available filter or by ultracentrifugation with 6% hetastarch. Reinfusion of white cells early during the reperfusion phase resulted in significantly increased pulmonary vascular resistance, airway pressure and lung edema, whereas minimal changes were seen when leukocytes were repleted after 60 minutes of reperfusion.[95,96] In a follow-up study in a bovine orthotopic heart-lung transplant model, the Johns Hopkins group demonstrated improved oxygen transfer following 12 hours of hypothermic storage when a leukocyte filter was incorporated into the extracorporeal circuit during organ procurement and at the time of transplantation.[97] A final experiment using the same model examined the role of combined treatment with leukocyte depletion and liposomal superoxide dismutase compared to either intervention alone in reducing reperfusion lung damage.[98] PO_2s after six hours of reperfusion were similar in the combined treatment and the leukocyte depletion groups, although the former exhibited less pulmonary edema and improved lung histology.

Despite the beneficial role of leukocyte depletion in these experiments, questions remain about the clinical applicability of this technique.[98] In order to profoundly deplete white cells from the allograft, use of a leukocyte filter would be necessary during both donor organ procurement and during graft implantation. This technique therefore has applicability only in the clinical setting of heart-lung transplantation, where donor core-cooling may be employed and the use of cardiopulmonary bypass in the recipient is mandatory. Ide and associates have reported beneficial effects of leukocyte depletion during warm lung ischemia and reperfusion in an in vivo canine model, using femoral artery and venous cannulation and in vivo blood filtration.[99] This technique, however, is too cumbersome for clinical use in lung transplantation. Furthermore, the uncertainty as to whether leukocyte depletion will result in increased postoperative infections[98] has prevented its

clinical application to date. A more practical approach might be the temporary modulation of the deleterious effects of white cells using corticosteroids and/or prostaglandins during organ procurement, and by the further use of corticosteroids and possibly inhibitors of the hydroxyl radical or other oxygen free radicals prior to and during reperfusion.

ALLOPURINOL

During ischemia the xanthine dehydrogenase enzyme is converted to xanthine oxidase.[86,100] Upon reperfusion, xanthine oxidase uses molecular oxygen as an electron acceptor, resulting in the formation of superoxide anions and other toxic oxygen radicals.[100] Allopurinol is a competitive inhibitor of the oxidase enzyme, and has been widely investigated in ischemia-reperfusion models in many organs, but only recently in experimental lung and heart-lung transplantation.

It has long been known that xanthine oxidase activity is lower in pigs and humans than in dogs.[101] This fact has raised questions concerning allopurinol's mechanism of action in the mitigation of ischemia-reperfusion injury. Although it is only a weak scavenger of the superoxide anion, allopurinol has been shown in vitro to facilitate electron transport, which could be beneficial during reperfusion when mitochondrial membrane lipids may be disordered.[100] Furthermore, allopurinol and its metabolite oxypurinol are potent scavengers of the very reactive hydroxyl free radical.[93,102] It is therefore likely that these substances exert their beneficial effects by virtue of a generalized upgrading of tissue anti-oxidant status rather than primarily by xanthine oxidase inhibition.[103]

To date, work from two institutions has investigated the role of allopurinol pretreatment of donor and recipient animals in lung transplantation. Bonser and associates, using a canine single lung autotransplant model, found optimal preservation after four hours of cold ischemia by the combination of allopurinol pretreatment and the perireperfusion administration of deferoxamine.[104] Unfortunately, the effect of allopurinol alone was not addressed in this study. Qayumi and associates have emphasized that the protective effect of allopurinol appears to be critically dependent on the nature of the pretreatment regimen, and that repeated allopurinol dosing for several days prior to the ischemic interval may be necessary for optimal effect.[103,105] In a swine orthotopic heart-lung transplant model, they noted a direct correlation between the functional viability of the transplanted lungs and the decrease in susceptibility of red blood cells from allpurinol-treated animals to in vitro oxidative challenge. Pigs with the greatest red cell anti-oxidant response following allopurinol treatment exhibited satisfactory cardiac and pulmonary function after six hours of ischemia; animals with a low red cell anti-oxidant activity developed a significantly higher lung water content and pulmonary vascular resistance, and a lower PO_2 during reperfusion. The authors concluded that measurement of erythrocyte susceptibility to in vitro oxidative challenge may prove useful in optimizing interventions prior to surgery in order to limit reperfusion injury.[103,105] Additional work is required using longer ischemic times to determine whether allopurinol therapy of lung recipients may be helpful in prolonged lung allograft preservation.

Deferoxamine

Over the past few years, much emphasis has been placed on the role of iron as a catalyst in the formation of the potent hydroxyl radical, and iron chelation with deferoxamine has been pursued especially in experimental renal[106] and cardiac[107,108] preservation. Deferoxamine has a low molecular weight, which may facilitate its intracellular penetration to the sites of free radical generation.[108] It not only counteracts hydroxyl radical formation via the Haber-Weiss reaction, but also inhibits the chain reactions of lipid peroxidation that occur during reperfusion injury.[107-109] Furthermore, deferoxamine is a direct scavenger of superoxide radicals, thus further mitigating free radical-mediated reperfusion damage.[110]

There have been relatively few studies on deferoxamine in the lung transplant literature. The beneficial effect of deferoxamine administered prior to and during reperfusion in a canine lung autotransplant model, in conjunction with allopurinol, has been noted above.[104] In rat single lung isografts stored for 48 hours after flushing with hypertonic citrate, deferoxamine failed to improve outcome.[111] Conversely, in a swine model of heart-lung transplantation, deferoxamine-treated recipients demonstrated superior lung function as compared to controls after four hours of hypothermic storage.[112]

Recently, Conte and associates studied the effect of deferoxamine treatment in canine left single lung transplantation, following 22 hours of $10°C$ preservation.[113] Deferoxamine was administered to donor and recipient dogs, and included in the pulmonary flush solution. Following right pulmonary artery ligation post-transplant, the deferoxamine group exhibited a significantly higher PO_2 and a lower pulmonary vascular resistance, which persisted throughout the six-hour reperfusion phase. The authors concluded that deferoxamine showed considerable promise in improving the long-term preservation of lung grafts.

Unlike other free radical scavengers, deferoxamine has been used clinically for years, in the treatment of iron and aluminum intoxication.[114] Its most commonly reported side effects include allergic reactions, gastrointestinal disturbances and tachycardia.[114] Recently, Hallaway and associates reported the synthesis of a new class of iron chelators, which were prepared by covalently attaching deferoxamine to biocompatible polymers such as dextran and hydroxyethyl-starch.[115] The iron binding properties of deferoxamine were unchanged after this procedure, but its plasma half-life was dramatically increased and its toxicity (in mice and dogs) markedly reduced. Further studies of the new complex deferoxamine derivatives are warranted in large animal lung transplant models, in view of the promising results already obtained with the free drug in the prolonged preservation of canine lung grafts.

Superoxide Dismutase and Catalase

The lung's endogenous defense mechanisms against free radical damage include the anti-oxidant enzymes superoxidase dismutase, catalase and glutathione peroxidase.[91,92] These enzymes may become depleted with prolonged ischemia or the burst of free radical generation on reperfusion may overwhelm the lung's native oxygen free radical-scavenging capabilities. Numerous experiments involving exogenous supplementation with superoxide dismutase and catalase have therefore been performed in an attempt to mitigate pulmonary reperfusion injury.

Several major theoretical objections have been raised concerning the use of exogenous superoxide dismutase in this setting. Firstly, superoxide dismutase has a relatively short plasma half-life of approximately 25 minutes in the dog after an intravenous bolus.[98] Secondly, superoxide dismutase is a protein, and is likely antigenic.[116] Thirdly, superoxide dismutase is a large molecule (molecular weight greater than 30,000 daltons) that would be expected to have a poor penetration into the cell.[85,98,116] Fortunately, the availability of a liposomal human recombinant superoxide dismutase preparation should decrease its antigenicity for human use and facilitate its access to intracellular sites.[28,98,117] Furthermore, although it has been assumed that superoxide radicals exert their deleterious effects only at the mitochondrial intracellular level,[116] Ratych and associates have demonstrated that the essential components for the production of free radicals during reperfusion exist within purified pulmonary endothelial cells.[118] This would permit exogenous superoxide dismutase to scavenge superoxide anions generated in the endothelial vascular network before the development of end-organ damage.[117]

Numerous studies since 1985 have confirmed the beneficial roles of superoxide dismutase and catalase in isolated, perfused lung models of ischemia-reperfusion injury.[84,85,88,89,119,120,121] Experiments in intact animal heart-lung transplant preparations have shown similar results.[28,98,117,122] In the latter group of experiments, free radical scavengers were usually administered during organ harvesting as well as during reperfusion. Recent work by Bando and associates, however, showed that superoxide dismutase was most effective in preventing reperfusion injury when

it was administered intravenously just prior to and at the onset of reperfusion.[117] These findings are consistent with the recent experiments by Paull and associates showing a marked attenuation of pulmonary reperfusion injury after 24 hours of hypothermic lung ischemia when superoxide dismutase and catalase were given upon the commencement of reperfusion.[85]

DIMETHYLTHIOUREA

It has long been known that thiourea compounds are efficient hydroxl radical scavengers in vitro, but their experimental use had been precluded by their tendency to cause fatal pulmonary edema in vivo.[123] In 1983 Fox and associates modified thiourea by N, N' dimethylation, and found that the dimethylthiourea derivative was nontoxic, while remaining a very potent hydroyxl radical scavenger.[123] Several years later, the University of North Carolina group began investigating dimethythiourea in hypothermic lung preservation in both isolated canine lobes[124] and in an in vivo dog single lung transplant model.[86,125,126]

Dimethylthiourea appears to offer several theoretical advantages over superoxide dismutase and catalase as an oxygen free radical scavenger for lung preservation.[124] It has a low molecular weight (104 daltons) and thus may enter cells readily. It is nonenzymatic and has a prolonged half-life of approximately 35 hours, which would be ideal in the setting of lung transplantation. Furthermore, dimethylthiourea directly counteracts the hydroxyl radical, which is probably the most destructive agent in oxidant lung injury.

Paull and associates have demonstrated that dimethylthiourea added to both the flush solution and reperfusate decreased pulmonary capillary permeability, as well as lung lipid peroxidation products, following four hours of cold storage.[124] A follow-up study using dimethylthiourea in the pulmonary flush solution only showed improved preservation in canine lobes stored at $4°C$ for 24 hours prior to transplantation.[125] Work by other investigators has confirmed that dimethylthiourea mitigates reperfusion injury in isolated rabbit[89] and dog[63] lungs following three hours of warm ischemia, but not in these same species after unilateral pulmonary artery snaring for 48 hours.[127]

Subsequent investigations by the University of North Carolina group have examined the effect of dimethylthiourea in a canine left lung transplant model, with ligation of the contralateral pulmonary artery and bronchus during reperfusion.[86,126] After 12 hours of 4°C preservation, dimethylthiourea-treated dogs exhibited a significantly better PO_2 and a lower pulmonary vascular resistance than nontreated controls during the first four to six hours of reperfusion.[126] After 24 hours of hypothermic storage, similar findings were noted in the early reperfusion phase, but lung function then worsened progressively and equally in both groups.[86] The authors postulated that this deterioration was due to the severe lung injury resulting from the 24-hour ischemic time, from which dimethylthiourea provided significant but only partial protection. Further work using dimethylthiourea in conjunction with other agents is indicated in an attempt to attenuate further reperfusion injury following prolonged preservation.

PLATELET-ACTIVATING FACTOR ANTAGONISTS

Recently, increasing attention has been directed to a phospholipid mediator of inflammatory reactions and ischemia-reperfusion injury that acts by a mechanism complementary to that of oxygen free radicals. This compound, first characterized as platelet-activating factor by Benveniste,[128] can be synthesized and released by white blood cells, macrophages, endothelial cells, and by platelets themselves.[129] Platelet-activating factor binds to a specific site on platelets, and is a potent inducer of platelet activation and aggregation.[129] Activated platelets are in turn capable of releasing potent mediators of inflammation such as bradykinin and other kinins through activated Hageman's factor.[129] In addition, platelet activating factor activates neutrophils, and triggers neutrophil aggregation, adherence, chemotaxis and degranulation.[130] The end result of these platelet-neutrophil interactions is the release of many inflammatory me-

diators, including leukotrienes, superoxide anions and eicosanoids that cause an increase in vascular permeability, altered vascular smooth muscle contractility and end-organ damage.[129]

Of interest in the setting of lung transplantation is the growing emphasis being placed on the role of platelet-activating factor in various lung injury states.[131-133] In addition, platelet-activating factor antagonists have been shown to mitigate hyperacute and cell-mediated graft rejection[134-136] and to improve the function of rat liver allografts after prolonged cold storage.[137] Multiple platelet-activating factor antagonists have been synthesized during the past six years,[138] and the potential role of these antagonists in lung preservation is being increasingly investigated.

Using a heterotopic heart-left lung transplant model in dogs, the Hannover group recently reported superior lung preservation following six hours of cold storage when the platelet activating factor antagonist WEB 2170 BS was infused during organ harvest as well as throughout reperfusion.[139] In a swine model of heart-lung transplantation, Qayumi and associates found improved heart and lung function post-transplant when the platelet activating factor antagonist CV-3988 was infused in recipient animals.[4] The Georgetown University group has had an interest in the platelet-activating factor antagonist BN 52021 for over five years. Recently, they investigated this antagonist in a canine model of left single lung transplantation, with flushing of the pulmonary artery with University of Wisconsin solution and donor and recipient treatment with BN 52021.[140] After six hours of hypothermic storage, BN 52021 was found to enhance lung preservation to a similar degree as deferoxamine. Most recently, the Georgetown University group examined the role of BN 52021 in extended lung graft preservation in dogs.[141] After 22 hours of 10°C storage, transplantation, and ligation of the contralateral pulmonary artery, the PO_2 in single lung grafts treated with BN 52021 was significantly higher and the pulmonary vascular resistance was significantly lower than in nontreated controls. The authors concluded that platelet-activating factor antagonists such as BN 52021 may be useful adjuncts in lung preservation. Further experiments using other potent platelet-activating factor antagonists alone or in combination with other agents that attenuate reperfusion lung injury are forthcoming.

SUMMARY

Over the past seven years considerable progress has been made in the understanding of the pathobiology of pulmonary ischemia-reperfusion injury and in the successful preservation of lung grafts for transplantation. It is evident that ischemia-reperfusion damage is a complex process which does not have a single etiology. Additional work needs to be done, especially in comprehending the multiple biochemical derangements that occur during the reperfusion phase, and in devising strategies to minimize reperfusion injury after prolonged ischemia. Furthermore, the standardization of experimental lung transplant models and the criteria by which lung preservation is assessed and reported by different investigators is mandatory if lung preservation research is to progress in an orderly manner. Over the past few years, official guidelines for reporting the performance of cardiac valve prostheses[142,143] and for interpreting endomyocardial[144] and transbronchial[145] biopsies have been published. Perhaps a consensus conference should be organized with the goal of standardizing data reporting in experimental lung preservation.

Almost all studies on experimental lung preservation to date have used lungs from normal animal donors. In the clinical situation, however, all lung grafts are compromised to some degree by aspiration, neurogenic pulmonary edema, trauma or sepsis prior to procurement. If the pool of donor lungs for clinical lung transplantation is to be significantly increased, techniques to "resuscitate" damaged lung grafts will need to be developed in the experimental laboratory. Perhaps by the time of the next review on lung preservation, reports on this topic will be forthcoming, and some of the newer advances in experimental lung preservation described in this review will have undergone successful clinical application.

ACKNOWLEDGEMENT

The authors thank Heather Motloch for her assistance in manuscript preparation and library research, and Dr. Fred Possmayer and Rudy Veldhuizen for their constructive review of this paper.

This chapter is reprinted with permission from Richard J. Novick. New trends in lung preservation: A collective review. J Heart and Lung Transplantation 1992. Copyright Mosby-Year Book, Inc.

REFERENCES

1. Haverich A, Scott WC, Jamieson SW. Twenty years of lung preservation - a review. J Heart Transplant 1985; 4:234-40.
2. Kaiser LR, Pasque MK, Trulock EP, Low DE, Dresler CM, Cooper JD. Bilateral sequential lung transplantation: The procedure of choice for double-lung replacement. Ann Thorac Surg 1991; 52:438-46.
3. Burdine J, Hertz MI, Snover DC, Bolman RM. Heart-lung and lung transplantation: Perioperative pulmonary dysfunction. Transplant Proc 1991; 23:1176-7.
4. Qayumi AK, Jamieson WRE, Poostizadeh A. Effect of platelet-activating factor antagonist CV-3988 in preservation of heart and lung for transplantation. Ann Thorac Surg 1991; 52:1026-32.
5. Wahlers T, Haverich A, Fieguth HG, Schafers HJ, Takayama T, Borst HG. Flush perfusion using Euro-Collins solution versus cooling by means of extracorporeal circulation in heart-lung preservation. J Heart Transplant 1986; 5:89-98.
6. Jurmann MJ, Dammenhayn L, Schafers HJ, Wahlers T, Fieguth HG, Haverich A. Prostacyclin as an additive to single crystalloid flush: Improved pulmonary preservation in heart-lung transplantation. Transplant Proc 1987; 19:4103-4.
7. Jones MT, Hsieh C, Yoshikwa K, Patterson GA, Cooper JD. A new model for assessment of lung preservation. J Thorac Cardiovasc Surg 1988; 96:608-14.
8. Keshavjee SH, Yamazaki F, Cardoso PF, McRitchie DI, Patterson GA, Cooper JD. A method for safe 12-hour pulmonary preservation. J Thorac Cardiovasc Surg 1989; 98:529-34.
9. Bonser RS, Fragomeni LS, Harris K et al. Acute physiologic changes after extended pulmonary preservation. J Heart Transplant 1990; 9:220-9.
10. Locke TJ, Hooper TL, Flecknell PA, McGregor CGA. Preservation of the lung: Comparison of topical cooling and cold crystalloid pulmonary perfusion. J Thorac Cardiovasc Surg 1988; 96:789-95.
11. Patterson GA, Mitzner WA, Sylvester JT. Assessment of fluid balance in isolated sheep lungs. J Appl Physiol 1985; 58:882-91.

12. LoCicero J, Massad M, Kamp D et al. Colloid versus crystalloid lung perfusion: Effect on leukocyte sequestration. Surg Forum 1989; 40:370-2.

13. LoCicero J, Massad M, Khasho FH, Matano J, Greene R, de Tarnowsky J. Sensitivity of aerodynamic changes for assessing pulmonary injury in the isolated perfused working lung model. Transplant Proc 1990; 22:559-60.

14. LoCicero J, Massad M, Matano J, Khasho F, Greene R. Aerodynamic evaluation of crystalloid and colloid flush perfusion for lung preservation. J Surg Res 1990; 49:469-75.

15. LoCicero J, Massad M, Matano J, Greene R, Dunn M, Michaelis LL. Contribution of the bronchial circulation to lung preservation. J Thorac Cardiovasc Surg 1991; 101:807-15.

16. LoCicero J, Massad M, Oba J, Greene R, de Tarnowsky J. Extended lung preservation by bronchial artery perfusion with University of Wisconsin solution. Transplant Proc 1991; 23:670-1.

17. Wang LS, Yoshikawa K, Miyoshi S et al. The effect of ishemic time and temperature on lung preservation in a simple *ex vivo* rabbit model used for functional assessment. J Thorac Cardiovasc Surg 1989; 98:333-42.

18. Yokomise H, Ueno T, Yamazaki F, Keshavjee S, Slutsky A, Patterson G. The effect and optimal time of administration of verapamil on lung preservation. Transplantation 1990; 49:1039-43.

19. Yamazaki F, Yokomise H, Keshavjee SH et al. The superiority of an extracellular fluid solution over Euro-Collins' solution for pulmonary preservation. Transplantation 1990; 49:690-4.

20. Weder W, Harper B, Shimokawa S et al. Influence of intraalveolar oxygen concentration on lung preservation in a rabbit model. J Thorac Cardiovasc Surg 1991; 101:1037-43.

21. Toronto Lung Transplant Group. Unilateral lung transplantation for pulmonary fibrosis. N Engl J Med 1986; 314:1140-5.

22. Hardesty RL, Griffith BP. Autoperfusion of the heart and lungs for preservation during distant procurement. J Thorac Cardiovasc Surg 1987; 93:11-9.

23. Yacoub MH, Khaghani A, Banner N, Tajkarimi S, Fitzgerald M. Distant organ procurement for heart and lung transplantation. Transplant Proc 1989; 21:2548-50.

24. Baumgartner WA, Williams GM, Fraser CD et al. Cardiopulmonary bypass with profound hypothermia: An optimal preservation method for multiorgan procurement. Transplantation 1989; 47:123-7.

25. Pillai R, Fraser C, Bando K, Brawn J, Reitz B, Baumgartner W. Core cooling remains the most effective technique of extended heart-lung preservation: Further experimental evidence. Transplant Proc 1990; 22:551-2.

26. Fraser CD, Tamura F, Adachi H et al. Donor core-cooling provides improved static preservation for heart-lung transplantation. Ann Thorac Surg 1988; 45:253-7.

27. Bando K, Teramoto S, Tago M et al. Core-cooling, heart-perfusion, lung-immersion technique provides successful cardiopulmonary preservation for heart-lung transplantation. Ann Thorac Surg 1988; 46:625-30.

28. Bando K, Teramoto S, Tago M, Teraoka H, Seno S, Senoo Y. Successful extended hypothermic cardiopulmonary preservation for heart-lung transplantation. J Thorac Cardiovasc Surg 1989; 98:137-46.

29. Harjula A, Baldwin JC, Shumway NE. Donor deep hypothermia or donor pretreatment with prostaglandin E1 and single pulmonary artery flush for heart-lung graft preservation: An experimental primate study. Ann Thorac Surg 1988; 46:553-5.

30. Locke TJ, Hooper TL, Flecknell PA, McGregor CGA. Preservation of the lung: Comparison of flush perfusion with cold modified blood and core cooling by cardiopulmonary bypass. J Heart Lung Transplant 1991; 10:1-8.

31. Haverich A, Wahlers T, Schafers HJ et al. Distant organ procurement in clinical lung- and heart-lung transplantation: Cooling by extracorporeal circulation or hypothermic flush. Eur J Cardio-thorac Surg 1990; 4:245-9.

32. Kirk AJB, Conacher ID, Corris PA, Dark JH. Single flush perfusion with Euro-Collins solution in lung preservation: Clinical assessment of early graft function. Transplant Proc 1990; 22:2238-9.

33. Starkey TD, Sakakibara N, Hagberg RC, Tazelaar HD, Baldwin JC, Jamieson SW. Successful six-hour cardiopulmonary preservation with simple hypothermic crystalloid flush. J Heart Transplant 1986; 5:291-7.

34. Haverich A, Aziz S, Scott WC, Jamieson SW, Shumway NE. Improved lung preservation using Euro-Collins solution for flush-perfusion. Thorac Cardiovasc Surg 1986; 34:368-76.

35. Baldwin JC, Frist WH, Starkey TD et al. Distant graft procurement for combined heart and lung transplantation using pulmonary artery flush and simple topical hypothermia for graft preservation. Ann Thorac Surg 1987; 43:670-3.

36. Jones KD, Cavarocchi N, Hakim M, Cory-Pearce R, English TAH, Wallwork J. A single flush technique for successful distant organ procurement in heart-lung transplantation. Heart Transplant 1985; 4:614.

37. Hakim M, Higenbottam T, Bethune D et al. Selection and procurement of combined heart and lung grafts for transplantation. J Thorac Cardiovasc Surg 1988; 95:474-9.

38. McGoldrick JP, Scott JP, Smyth R, Higenbottam T, Wallwork J. Early graft function after heart-lung transplantation. J Heart Transplant 1990; 9:693-8.

39. Hooper TL, Locke TJ, Fetherston G, Flecknell PA, McGregor CGA. Comparison of cold flush perfusion with modified blood versus modified Euro-Collins solution for lung preservation. J Heart Transplant 1990; 9:429-34.

40. Fujimura S, Kondo T, Handa M et al. Successful 24-hour preservation of canine lung transplants using modified extracellular fluid. Transplant Proc 1985; 17:1466-7.

41. Fujimura S, Handa M, Kondo T, Ichinose T, Shiraishi Y, Nakada T. Successful 48-hour simple hypothermic perfusion of canine lung transplants. Transplant Proc 1987; 19:1334-6.

42. Unruh H, Hoppensack M, Oppenheimer L. Vascular properties of canine lungs perfused with Eurocollins solution and prostacyclin. Ann Thorac Surg 1990; 49:292-8.

43. Puskas JD, Cardoso PFG, Mayer E, Shi S, Slutsky AS, Patterson GA. Equivalent 18-hour lung preservation by pulmonary flush with low potassium dextran or Euro-Collins solution after prostaglandin E1 infusion. J Thorac Cardiovasc Surg1992; 104:83-9.

44. Jamieson NV, Sundberg R, Lindell S et al. Preservation of the canine liver for 24-48 hours using simple cold storage with UW solution. Transplantation 1988; 46:517-22.

45. Ploeg RJ, Goossens D, McAnulty JF, Southard JH, Belzer FO. Successful 72-hour cold storage of dog kidneys with UW solution. Transplantation 1988; 46:191-6.

46. Wahlberg JA, Love R, Landegaard L, Southard JH, Belzer FO. Seventy-two hour preservation of the canine pancreas. Transplantation 1987; 43:5-8.

47. Kalayoglu M, Stratta RJ, Sollinger HW et al. Clinical results in liver transplantation using UW solution for extended preservation. Transplant Proc 1989; 21:1342-3.

48. Semik M, Moller F, Lange V, Bernhard A, Toomes H. Comparison of Euro-Collins and UW-1 solutions for lung preservation using the parabiotic rat perfusion model. Transplant Proc 1990; 22:2235-6.

49. Kawahara K, Ikari H, Hisano H et al. Twenty-four hour canine lung preservation using UW solution. Transplantation 1991; 51:584-7.

50. Naka Y, Shirakura R, Matsuda H et al. Canine heart-lung transplantation after 24-hour hypothermic preservation. Eur J Cardio-Thorac Surg 1990; 4:499-503.

51. Naka Y, Shirakura R, Matsuda H et al. Canine heart-lung transplantation after 24-hour hypothermic preservation with Belzer-UW solution. J Heart Lung Transplant 1991; 10:296-303.

52. Rinaldi M, Nilsson FN, Locke TJ, Spackman TN, McGregor CGA. Successful 24-hour preservation of the canine lung with UW-lactobionate solution. J Heart Lung Transplant 1991; 10:158.

53. Moen J, Claesson K, Pienaar H et al. Preservation of dog liver, kidney, and pancreas using the Belzer-UW solution with a high-sodium and low-potassium content. Transplantation 1989; 47:940-5.

54. Oka T, Puskas JD, Mayer E et al. Low potassium UW solution for lung preservation: Comparison with regular UW, LPD and Euro-Collins' solutions. Transplantation1991; 52:984-8.

55. Jamieson NV, Lindell S, Sundberg R, Southard JH, Belzer FO. An analysis of the components in UW solution using the isolated perfused rabbit liver. Transplantation 1988; 46:512-6.

56. Wicomb WN, Collins GM. Twenty-four hour rabbit heart storage with UW solution. Transplantation 1989; 48:6-9.

57. Astier A, Paul M. Instability of reduced glutathione in commerical Belzer cold storage solution. Lancet 1989; 2:556-7.

58. Wolkowicz PE, Caulfield JB. Cardioplegia with aged UW solution induces loss of cardiac collagen. Transplantation 1991; 51:898-901.

59. Novick RJ, Reid KR, Denning L, Duplan J, Menkis AH, McKenzie FN. Prolonged preservation of canine lung allografts: the role of prostaglandins. Ann Thorac Surg 1991; 51:853-9.

60. Hooper TL, Fetherston GJ, Flecknell PA, Dark JH, McGregor CGA. The use of a prostacyclin analog, Iloprost, as an adjunct to pulmonary preservation with Euro-Collins solution. Transplantation 1990; 49:495-9.

61. Bonser RS, Fragomeni LS, Jamieson SW et al. Effects of prostaglandin E_1 in 12-hour lung preservation. J Heart Lung Transplant 1991; 10:310-6.

62. Weiss SJ. Tissue destruction by neutrophils. N Engl J Med 1989; 320:365-76.

63. Matsumura A, Nakahara K, Miyoshi S, Mizuta T, Akashi A, Kawashima Y. Filtration coefficient in isolated preserved and reperfused canine lung. J Surg Res 1991; 50:205-11.

64. Hammerschmidt DE, White JG, Craddock PR, Jacob HS. Corticosteroids inhibit complement-induced granulocyte aggregation: A possible mechanism for their efficacy in shock states. J Clin Invest 1979; 63:798-803.

65. Hall TS, Borkon AM, Gurtner GC et al. Improved static lung preservation with corticosteroids and hypothermia. J Heart Tranplant 1988; 7:348-52.

66. Hooper TL, Jones MT, Thomson DS et al. Modulation of ischemic lung injury by corticosteroids. Transplantation 1990; 50:530-2.

67. Cheung JY, Bonventre JV, Malis CD, Leaf A. Calcium and ischemic injury. N Engl J Med 1986; 314:1670-6.

68. Fuller BJ, Gower JD, Green CJ. Free radical damage and organ preservation: fact or fiction? A review of the interrelationship between oxidative stress and physiological ion disbalance. Cryobiology 1988; 25:377-93.

69. Hachida M, Morton DL. The protection of ischemic lung with verapamil and hydralazine. J Thorac Cardiovasc Surg 1988; 95:178-83.

70. Hachida M, Morton DL. A new solution (UCLA formula) for lung preservation. J Thorac Cardiovasc Surg 1989; 97:513-20.

71. Hachida M, Morton DL. Lung function after prolonged lung preservation. J Thorac Cardiovasc Surg 1989; 97:911-9.

72. Karck M, Schmid C, Siclari F, Dammenhayn L, Haverich A. Effects of calcium channel blockage in postischemic lung reperfusion. Transplant Proc 1990; 22:2237.

73. Deffebach ME, Charan NB, Lakshminarayan S, Butler J. The bronchial circulation: Small, but a vital attribute of the lung. Am Rev Respir Dis 1987; 135:463-81.

74. Blades B, Pierpont HC, Samadi A, Hill RP. The

effect of experimental lung ischemia on pulmonary function. Surg Forum 1953; 4:255-60.

75. Veith FJ, Sinha SBP, Graves JS, Boley SJ, Dougherty JC. Ischemic tolerance of the lung: Effect of ventilation and inflation. J Thorac Cardiovasc Surg 1971; 61:804-10.

76. Joseph WL, Morton DL. Influence of ischemia and hypothermia on the ability of the transplanted primate lung to provide immediate and total respiratory support. J Thorac Cardiovasc Surg 1971; 62:752-62.

77. Kondo Y, Turner MD, Cockrell JV, Hardy JD. Ischemic tolerance of the canine autotransplanted lung. Surgery 1974; 76:447-53.

78. Ueno T, Yokomise H, Oka T et al. The effect of PgE$_1$ and temperature on lung function following preservation. Transplantation 1991; 52:626-30.

79. Shimokawa S, Watanabe S, Uehara K, Taira A. A new lung preservation method of topical cooling by ambient cold air: An experimental study. Transplant Proc 1991; 23:653-4.

80. Okaniwa G, Nakada T, Kawakami M et al. Studies on the preservation of canine lung at subzero temperatures. J Thorac Cardiovasc Surg 1973; 65:180-6.

81. Kon ND, Hines MH, Harr CD et al. Improved lung preservation with cold air storage. Ann Thorac Surg 1991; 51:557-62.

82. Cooper JD, Pearson FG, Patterson GA et al. Technique of successful lung transplantation in humans. J Thorac Cardiovasc Surg 1987; 93:173-81.

83. Puskas JD, Hirai T, Christie N, Mayer E, Slutsky AS, Patterson GA. Reliable 30-hour lung preservation by donor hyperinfation. J Thorac Cardiovasc Surg 1992; 104:1075-83.

84. Koyama I, Toung TJK, Rogers MC, Gurtner GH, Traystman RJ. O2 radicals mediate reperfusion lung injury in ischemic O2-ventilated canine pulmonary lobe. J Appl Physiol 1987; 63:111-5.

85. Paull DE, Keagy BA, Kron EJ, Wilcox BR. Reperfusion injury in the lung preserved for 24 hours. Ann Thorac Surg 1989; 47:187-92.

86. Detterbeck FC, Keagy BA, Paull DE, Wilcox BR. Oxygen free radical scavengers decrease reperfusion injury in lung transplantation. Ann Thorac Surg 1990; 50:204-10.

87. Ljungman AG, Grum CM, Deeb GM, Bolling SF, Morganroth ML. Inhibition of cyclooxygenase metabolite production attenuates ischemia-reperfusion lung injury. Am Rev Respir Dis 1991; 143:610-7.

88. Kennedy T, Rao N, Hopkins C, Tolley E, Hoidal J. Reperfusion injury occurs in the lung by free radical mechanisms. Chest 1988; 93:149S.

89. Kennedy TP, Rao NV, Hopkins C, Pennington L, Tolley E, Hoidal JR. Role of reactive oxygen species in reperfusion injury of the rabbit lung. J Clin Invest 1989; 83:1326-35.

90. McCord JM, Fridovich I. The biology and pathology of oxygen radicals. Ann Intern Med 1978; 89:122-7.

91. Frank L, Massaro D. Oxygen toxicity. Am J Med 1980; 69:117-26.

92. Deneke SM, Fanburg BL. Normobaric oxygen toxicity of the lung. N Engl J Med 1980; 303:76-86.

93. Tabayashi K, Suzuki Y, Nagamine S, Ito Y, Sekino Y, Mohri H. A clinical trial of allopurinol (Zyloric) for myocardial protection. J Thorac Cardiovasc Surg 1991; 101:713-8.

94. Steinberg H, Greenwald RA, Sciubba J, Das DK. The effect of oxygen-derived free radicals on pulmonary endothelial cell function in the isolated perfused rat lung. Exp Lung Res 1982; 3:163-73.

95. Breda MA, Hall TS, Stuart RS et al. Twenty-four hour lung preservation by hypothermia and leukocyte depletion. Heart Transplant 1985; 4:325-9.

96. Hall TS, Breda MA, Baumgartner WA et al. The role of leukocyte depletion in reducing injury to the lung after hypothermic ischemia. Curr Surg 1987; 44:137-9.

97. Pillai R, Bando K, Schueler S, Zebley M, Reitz BA, Baumgartner WA. Leukocyte depletion results in excellent heart-lung function after 12 hours of storage. Ann Thorac Surg 1990; 50:211-4.

98. Bando K, Schueler S, Cameron DE et al. Twelve-hour cardiopulmonary preservation using donor core cooling, leukocyte depletion, and liposomal superoxide dismutase. J Heart Lung Transplant 1991; 10:304-9.

99. Ide H, Ino T, Hasegawa T, Matsumoto H. The role of leukocyte depletion by in vivo use of leukocyte filter in lung preservation after warm ischemia. Angiology 1990; 41:318-27.

100. Peterson DA, Kelly B, Gerrard JM. Allopurinol can act as an electron transfer agent: Is this relevant during reperfusion injury? Biochem Biophys Res Commun 1986; 137:76-9.

101. al-Khalidi UAS, Chaglassian TH. The species distribution of xanthine oxidase. Biochem J 1965; 97:318-20.

102. Moorhouse PC, Grootveld M, Halliwell B, Quinlan JG, Gutteridge JMC. Allopurinol and oxypurinol are hydroxyl radical scavengers. FEBS Lett 1987; 213:23-8.

103. Qayumi AK, Jamieson WRE, Godin DV et al. Response to allopurinol pretreatment in a swine model of heart-lung transplantation. J Invest Surg 1990; 3:331-40.

104. Bonser RS, Fragomeni LS, Edwards BJ et al. Allopurinol and deferroxamine improve canine lung preservation. Transplant Proc 1990; 22:557-8.

105. Godin DV, Ko KM, Qayumi AK, Jamieson WRE. A method for monitoring the effectiveness of allopurinol pretreatment in the prevention of ischemic/reperfusion injury. J Pharmacol Methods 1989; 22:289-97.

106. Fuller BJ, Lunec J, Healing G, Simpkin S, Green CJ. Reduction of susceptibility to lipid peroxidation by desferrioxamine in rabbit kidneys subjected to 24-hour cold ischemia and reperfusion. Transplantation 1987; 43:604-6.

107. Menasche P, Grousset C, Gauduel Y, Mouas C, Piwnica A. Prevention of hydroxyl radical formation: a critical concept for improving cardioplegia. Protective effects of deferoxamine. Circulation 1987; 76 (suppl V), V-180 - 5.

108. Menasche P, Grousset C, Mouas C, Piwnica A. A promising approach for improving the recovery of heart transplants: prevention of free radical injury through iron chelation by deferoxamine. J Thorac Cardiovasc Surg 1990; 100:13-21.

109. Aust SD, Morehouse LA, Thomas CE. Role of metals in oxygen radical reactions. J Free Radicals Biol Med 1985; 1:3-25.

110. Sinaceur J, Ribiere C, Nordmann J, Nordmann R. Desferrioxamine: A scavenger of superoxide radicals? Biochem Pharmacol 1984; 33:1693-4.

111. Pickford MA, Gower JD, Simpkin S, Sampson M, Green CJ. Function of single rat lung isografts after 48-hour cold storage: The effect of treatment with free radical antagonists and prostacyclin PGI_2. Transplantation 1991; 51:743-9.

112. Qayumi AK, Jamieson WRE, Poostizadeh A, Germann E, Gillespie KD. Comparison of new iron chelating agents in the prevention of ischemia/reperfusion injury-a swine model of heart-lung transplantation. J Invest Surg (in press).

113. Conte JV, Katz NM, Foegh ML, Wallace RB, Ramwell PW. Iron chelation therapy and lung transplantation: Effects of deferoxamine on lung preservation in canine single lung transplantation. J Thorac Cardiovasc Surg 1991; 101:1024-9.

114. Klassen CD. Heavy metals and heavy-metal antagonists. In: Gilman AG, Rall TW, Nies AS, Taylor P, eds. The Pharmacological Basis of Therapeutics. New York: Pergamon Press, 1990:1611-2.

115. Hallaway PE, Eaton JW, Panter SS, Hedlund BE. Modulation of deferoxamine toxicity and clearance by covalent attachment to biocompatible polymers. Proc Natl Acad Sci USA 1989; 86:10108-12.

116. McKenzie FN, in discussion of Reichart BA, Novitzky D, Cooper DKC, Cunningham MS, Rose AG. Successful orthotopic heart-lung transplantation in the baboon after five hours of cold ischemia with cardioplegia and Collins' solution. J Heart Transplant 1987; 6:15-22.

117. Bando K, Tago N, Teraoka H, Seno S, Senoo Y, Teramoto S. Extended cardiopulmonary preservation for heart-lung transplantation: A comparative study of superoxide dismutase. J Heart Transplant 1989; 8:59-66.

118. Ratych RE, Chuknyiska RS, Bulkley GB. The primary localization of free radical generation after anoxia/reoxygenation in isolated endothelial cells. Surgery 1987; 102:122-31.

119. Stuart RS, Baumgartner WA, Borkon AM et al. Five-hour hypothermic lung preservation with oxygen-free radical scavengers. Transplant Proc 1985; 17:1454-6.

120. Grosso MA, Brown JM, Viders DE et al. Xanthine oxidase-derived oxygen radicals induce pulmonary edema by direct endothelial cell injury. J Surg Res 1989; 46:355-60.

121. Takayama T, Auerswald A, Schafers HJ, Dammenhayn L, Haverich A. The protective effect of superoxide dismutase during reperfusion of the ischemic lung. Transplant Proc 1987; 19:1332-3.

122. Cremer J, Jurmann M, Dammenhayn L, Wahlers T, Haverich A, Borst HG. Oxygen free radical scavengers to prevent pulmonary reperfusion injury after heart-lung transplantation. J Heart Transplant 1989: 8:330-6.

123. Fox RB, Harada RN, Tate RM, Repine JE. Prevention of thiourea-induced pulmonary edema by hydroxyl-radical scavengers. J Appl Physiol 1983; 55:1456-9.

124. Paull DE, Keagy BA, Kron EJ, Wilcox BR. Improved lung preservation using a dimethylthiourea flush. J Surg Res 1989; 46:333-8.

125. Paull DE, Padyk P, Kron E, Keagy BA, Wilcox BR. Dimethylthiourea flush improves transplant lung function following 24-hour cold preservation. Curr Surg 1989; 46:293-5.

126. Lambert CJ, Egan TM, Detterbeck FC, Keagy BA, Wilcox BR. Enhanced pulmonary function using dimethylthiourea for twelve-hour lung preservation. Ann Thorac Surg 1991; 51:924-30.

127. Bishop MJ, Chi EY, Su M, Cheney FW. Dimethylthiourea does not ameliorate reperfusion injury in dogs or rabbits. J Appl Physiol 1988; 65:2051-6.

128. Benveniste J, Henson PM, Cochrane CG. Leukocyte-dependent histamine release from rabbit platelets: The role of IgE, basophils and a platelet-activating factor. J Exp Med 1972; 136:1356-77.

129. Benveniste J, Chignard M. A role for PAF-acether (platelet-activating factor) in platelet-dependent vascular diseases? Circulation 1985; 72:713-7.

130. Shaw JO, Pinckard RN, Ferrigni KS, McManus LM, Hanahan DJ. Activation of human neutrophils with 1-O-hexadecyl/octadecyl-2-acetyl-sn-glyceryl-3-phosphorylcholine (platelet activating factor). J Immunol 1981; 127:1250-5.

131. Coyle AJ, Page CP. The role of PAF in pulmonary pathology. In: Handley DA, Saunders RN, Houlihan WJ, Tomesch JC, eds. Platelet-Activating Factor in Endotoxin and Immune Diseases. New York: Marcel Dekker, Inc., 1990:285-306.

132. Christman BW, Snapper JR. Role of PAF in endotoxin-induced lung dysfunction. In: Handley DA, Saunders RN, Houlihan WJ, Tomesch JC, eds. Platelet-Activating Factor in Endotoxin and Immune Diseases. New York: Marcel Dekker, Inc., 1990:497-518.

133. Chang SW, Voelkel NF. The role of platelet-activating factor in endotoxic shock and lung injury. In: Handley DA, Saunders RN, Houlihan WJ, Tomesch JC, eds. Platelet-Activating Factor in Endotoxin and Immune Diseases. New York: Marcel Dekker, Inc., 1990:629-54.

134. Foegh ML, Khirabadi BS, Rowles JR, Braquet P, Ramwell PW. Prolongation of cardiac allograft survival with BN 52021, a specific antagonist of platelet-activating factor. Transplantation 1986; 42:86-8.

135. Foegh ML, Hartmann DP, Rowles JR et al. Leukotrienes, thromboxane, and platelet activating factor in organ transplantation. Adv Prostaglandin Thromboxane Leukotriene Res 1987; 17:140-6.

136. Foegh ML, Chambers E, Khirabadi BS, Nakanishi

T, Ramwell PW. Platelet-activating factor in organ transplant rejection. Adv Prostaglandin Thrombaxane Leukotriene Res 1989; 19:377-82.

137. Ontell SJ, Makowka L, Boccagni P, Starzl TE. The role of PAF and its antagonism in transplantation: organ ischemia and preservation. In: Handley DA, Saunders RN, Houlihan WJ, Tomesch JC, eds. Platelet-Activating Factor in Endotoxin and Immune Diseases. New York: Marcel Dekker, Inc., 1990:419-47.

138. Houlihan WJ. Platelet-activating factor antagonists. In: Handley DA, Saunders RN, Houlihan WJ, Tomesch JC, eds. Platelet-Activating Factor in Endotoxin and Immune Diseases. New York: Marcel Dekker, Inc., 1990:31-75.

139. Wahlers T, Hirt S, Fieguth HG, Jurmann M, Haverich A, Borst HG. Future horizons of lung preservation by application of PAF-antagonists compared to current clinical standard (Euro-Collins flush-perfusion versus donor core cooling by extracorporeal circulation). J Thorac Cardiovasc Surg (in press).

140. Corcoran PC, Wang Y, Katz NM et al. Platelet activating factor antagonist enhances lung preserva- tion in a canine model of single lung allo- transplantation. J Thorac Cardiovasc Surg 1992; 104:66-72.

141. Conte JV, Katz NM, Wallace RB, Foegh ML. Long- term lung preservation with the PAF antagonist BN 52021. Transplantation 1991; 51:1152-6.

142. Weisel RD, Miller DC. Guidelines for reporting the performance of cardiac valve prostheses. CardiacSurgery: State of the Art Reviews. Philadelphia:Hanley & Belfus, Inc., 1987; 1:159-70.

143. Edmunds LH, Clark RE, Cohn LH, Miller DC, Weisel RD. Guidelines for reporting morbidity and mortality after cardiac valvular operations. Ann Thorac Surg 1988; 46:257-61.

144. Billingham ME, Cary NRB, Hammond ME, et al. A working formulation for the standardization of no- menclature and the diagnosis of heart and lung rejection: heart rejection study group. J Heart Trans- plant 1990;9:587-93.

145. Yousem SA, Berry GJ, Brunt EM et al. A working formulation for the standardization of nomenclature in the diagnosis of heart and lung rejection: Lung rejection study group. J Heart Transplant 1990; 9:593-601.

INDEX